The
WITCH'S
Guide to
WELLNESS

The
WITCH'S
Guide to
WELLNESS

Natural, Magical Ways
to Treat, Heal, and Honor
Your Body, Mind, and Spirit

KRYSTLE L. JORDAN
Foreword by Arin Murphy-Hiscock,
Author of *The Witch's Book of Self-Care*

ADAMS MEDIA
NEW YORK   LONDON   TORONTO   SYDNEY   NEW DELHI

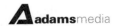

Adams Media
An Imprint of Simon & Schuster, Inc.
100 Technology Center Drive
Stoughton, Massachusetts 02072

First Adams Media hardcover edition
March 2022

ADAMS MEDIA and colophon are
trademarks of Simon & Schuster.

For information about special
discounts for bulk purchases, please
contact Simon & Schuster Special
Sales at 1-866-506-1949 or
business@simonandschuster.com.

The Simon & Schuster Speakers Bureau
can bring authors to your live event. For
more information or to book an event
contact the Simon & Schuster Speakers
Bureau at 1-866-248-3049 or visit our
website at www.simonspeakers.com.

Interior design by Julia Jacintho
Images © Creative Market/Pixejoo;
123RF/Oksana Tsvyk, perori

Manufactured in the
United States of America

1 2022

Library of Congress Cataloging-in-
Publication Data
Names: Jordan, Krystle L., author. |
Murphy-Hiscock, Arin, other.
Title: The witch's guide to wellness /
Krystle L. Jordan; foreword by Arin
Murphy-Hiscock, author of The Witch's
Book of Self-Care.
Description: First Adams Media hardcover
edition. | Stoughton, Massachusetts: Adams
Media, 2022. | Includes index.
Identifiers: LCCN 2021047285 |
ISBN 9781507217931 (hc) |
ISBN 9781507217948 (ebook)
Subjects: LCSH: Witchcraft. | Magic. |
Naturopathy.
Classification: LCC BF1566 .J677 2022 |
DDC 203/.3--dc23/eng/20211102
LC record available at https://lccn.loc
.gov/2021047285

ISBN 978-1-5072-1793-1
ISBN 978-1-5072-1794-8 (ebook)

This book is dedicated to my incredible wife, Thania, for always believing in me and encouraging me to persevere and follow my dreams. You are my love, my light, my magic.

Acknowledgments

Many thanks to my team at Adams Media for giving me this incredible opportunity and trusting me with this title—especially to Julia, for your positivity and immense support throughout the entire process, and to Brett for being an insightful, to-the-point editor. This book is what it is thanks to your knowledge and guidance.

I also have to thank my brilliant and beautiful wife, Thania, for reading every word I wrote and offering your own unique thoughts and perspective. Without you, this book may have never gotten finished! And thank you also to my wonderful son, Caedmon, for being patient and understanding when I was at my computer all day long. I love you infinitely.

A mention must be made to the book that solidified my journey as a witch, *Merlin's Book of Magick and Enchantment* by Nevill Drury. It spoke to me in a way no book ever had, and I knew I was on the right path.

Lastly, to everyone who has purchased this book, thank you! It's been a true honor to write, and I hope it is as therapeutic to you as writing it has been for me.

Contents

CHAPTER FOUR
Magic for Mental and Emotional Wellness.............. 141

◄◄◄~

CHAPTER FIVE
Magic for
Spiritual Wellness 193

Foreword

People often assume that magic affects things apart from a witch, or that it's used to shape the world to the witch's desire. This belief couldn't be further from the truth.

Magic is one of your most powerful tools for working to improve your own well-being—spiritually, emotionally, and mentally. It's not grand, sweeping change, either. It's small, incremental shifts that bring you closer to harmony within yourself. And when you have balance within yourself, it's easier to move in harmony with the world around you.

The two things that you can most effectively control and affect are yourself and your energy. In a world where we are continually buffeted by people, environment, and situations, cultivating awareness of your energy and fine-tuning it for optimal wellness is an act of self-care.

Even small actions add up. Maintenance is, after all, one of the keys to wellness. Regular maintenance on a car catches problems before they can strand you at the side of the road. The same goes for your personal wellness. Working to stay in tune with your needs on a regular basis enables you to become familiar with rhythms and tides within your life. That familiarity allows you to become aware of minor changes so that you can address them before they need a more significant investment of time and energy to remedy.

Infusing your daily activities with spiritual awareness will help you create a magical environment that fosters your spiritual, mental, and emotional health. For example, adjusting or updating the energy of your home helps maximize the positive and supportive energy surrounding you; weaving cleansings, blessings, and affirmations into your daily life enriches your connection to the energy surrounding you, encouraging gratitude and a positive outlook; and releasing things you no longer need or emotions that do not support spiritual wellness frees you from energy drain.

Working to nourish your body, mind, and spirit in daily life makes for optimal balance and living. Caring for all aspects of yourself improves your quality of life. Balancing and maintaining your personal energy also makes you better able to manage energy (yours and the energy you raise) in ritual and spell work. It also improves your connection to the natural world, which is always a bonus for a witch.

In this wonderful collection of spells, rituals, meditations, and affirmations, Krystle provides you with the magical tools to address imbalances in many different aspects of your life, for various situations. Most are small, easy ways to adjust your energy and encourage awareness within yourself. They can be easily added into your routines, or called on when required to apply to specific situations or problems.

Maintaining your holistic wellness makes you stronger, more resilient, and more able to deal with change. It's a gift to yourself, and an act of self-love. Take the time to tend to your wellness. It's an investment in yourself, and your spiritual path.

Introduction

Your path to wellness is an organic, evolving journey of art and magic.

Magic grants you strength, confidence, and a connection to something greater than yourself—but it can also help heal you from within. Just as you use magic to shift energies to create desirable changes in your life, you can also use its power to infuse your body and mind with strength and well-being. When you begin to shift the energies of your body, mind, and spirit, positive change will begin to take place.

The Witch's Guide to Wellness will help you build and grow your most magical and thriving self. Wellness is a journey, and it takes the same focus, patience, and creativity as your magical practice. In fact, the two are intertwined: As you deepen your understanding of how to make your physical and mental selves stronger and more resilient, you'll find you gain insight into your practice and how to develop and grow spiritually as well.

Within these pages, you will find more than 135 transformative practices that will help unite your witchcraft and wellness paths. There are rituals that will strengthen your physical body through movement; magical whole-food recipes that will nourish you, body and soul; practices to tune in to your innate power; exercises to draw your thoughts inward for self-reflection; herbal remedies to boost physical and emotional healing; and much more.

Taking care of your body, mind, and spirit is an act of love and reverence for yourself, the world around you, and for your magical path. Allowing your magic to shine a light on your wellness will enable your whole self to transition to a higher realm of possibility and begin feeling your absolute best: physically, mentally, spiritually, and magically. Let this book be the first step toward a beautiful transformation that will have you feeling magical, healthy, and present every single day.

CHAPTER ONE

Introduction to Magical Wellness

Blending your spiritual path, your magic, and your body's well-being in a harmonious journey can be a challenging and incredibly rewarding quest. When you're at your best physically and mentally, your spirit and magic benefit greatly, and vice versa: When your spiritual and magical realms are strong, your physical and mental selves thrive. This synergy builds dynamic inner connections—connections capable of creating incredible magic within yourself.

Wellness may seem like a modern concept, but it certainly isn't. For millennia, humans have prepared tinctures and potions and used crystal healing as a means to better health and longer life. But what exactly is wellness and how can it relate to your magical practice? This chapter will explore what wellness is and the relationship it has with your magical practice, as well as how to tailor your magical wellness practice to your needs and how to connect to your inner magic to start a magical wellness journey.

Witchcraft and Wellness:
Rooted in Ancient Knowledge

Witches have long been associated with healing. They were the ones with wisdom of the earth and all of its beautiful and mysterious secrets, the ones that knew a remedy for an upset stomach as well as a broken heart, and the ones intimately connected to the incredible world of nature that surrounds us. Even in the modern world, this remains true. Those who take on a nature-based spiritual path are often more in tune with and mindful of not only the natural world but of themselves. They embrace the healing properties of plants and herbs, they are familiar with the magical energies of the elements, they work with the seasons and rhythms of the land, and they know that truly being well extends beyond the physical body to the spirit.

Centuries before modern medicine, people turned to magic, potions, prayer, ritual, the properties of herbs, and the movement of the stars to aid, heal, and achieve this elusive state of wellness. Witches learned, tried, and tested natural remedies with wisdom and dedication; they were the healers, the midwives, and the wise ones. They pulled their healing power from the earth, shaped it, and utilized it for the good of others.

Witches held knowledge and power that was threatening to the upper class and, later, the emerging medical profession. Especially during the Early Modern Era (from around the mid-fifteenth century through the eighteenth century), witches were persecuted for a number of accusations, including not only harming but healing as well. Even "good witches" were marked by persecutors as needing to be wiped from the land. Though the negative stigma around the word "witch" has changed, it still exists today. It's time to take back that power, take on that lineage and ancient healing knowledge, then learn to shape, shift, and integrate your magic into your own wellness.

What Is Wellness?

Wellness consists of the lifestyle choices you implement each day to have your whole self—body, mind, and spirit—functioning at its highest level. Wellness, like magic, is not a static state but is ever changing and evolving, like the energy that is constantly taking new shape all around you. Wellness means taking action, accepting responsibility for yourself, nurturing your inner magic, and striving each day to move toward an overall healthier holistic self.

You want to live your life feeling radiant and relaxed, avoiding illness, being full of energy, and moving through your days like the ethereal spirit that you are. Feeling this way, however, is often elusive—there is nothing simple about shaping your wellness journey. In reality, things get in the way, some things are out of your control, and even when you have the best of intentions, your wellness, and sometimes your magic, often don't take top priority.

So, what's missing? What could be that one thing that pushes you to finally reach a point of total wellness? It might just be a bit of magic. From setting intentions with your morning beverage to enchanting your jewelry and embracing the powerful properties of plants, the magic of the universe surrounds you. Allow this magic to be the key to taking control of your wellness and your life.

Uniting Your Magic and Wellness

Whether you're aware of it or not, your magic is already an integral part of your overall well-being. Your magic can heal you, enrich you, and help shape you into your most inspired and unique self. Your magical practice provides insight into your emotional self, gives your body a lovely shot of endorphins (happy hormones) when you perform spell work, helps heal you physically by aligning the body systems, and alleviates stress when moving through meditations.

When you combine your magic and wellness practice, you'll notice incredible transformations begin to manifest within you. You'll be waking up energetic, motivated, and centered, and your ritual work will be stronger than ever. Utilizing your practice in this way empowers you to take control of your health, wellness, and healing path. This instills a sense of confidence and knowledge that you are in control of your journey and wellness. While you should always seek out a medical professional when you are ill, doing all that you can in your daily life to feel your best is allowing yourself to have the power: the power of action, the power of positivity, the power of your own personal brand of magic. Acknowledging and embracing this power will set you up for holistic wellness and magical success.

Accepting magic into your wellness journey is a crucial step to aligning your body, mind, and spirit. Doing so will allow new pathways to open, deepening the connections among your personal power, inner strength, and the earth. As you use magic to shift energies, you will create balance, clear away negativity, ignite happiness, achieve inner peace, and find confidence. It's time to start breaking the chains of old patterns and welcoming in new ways of being and of directing your magic. Welcome the beautiful energy of the tree outside your window, the strength of all four elements, the majestic power of the moon, and the vast knowledge of the universe; welcome them and use them to enhance your own witch potential, magical abilities, and overall health.

As a witch, you have an abundance of resources at your disposal such as spell work, crystals (also called "stones"), and herb knowledge, but the most important resource is what you already have inside: that strength, awareness, intuition, and resilience. It's all there waiting to be found. Use your magical practice to help nurture and liberate these pieces of you. Choose your crystals with awareness and purpose, embody your connection to nature, use the strength of your spoken words to manifest and grow, perform shadow work to move past pain, and learn to trust your intuition. All these actions work together so that you may feel centered, discover new things about yourself, let go of old wounds, and deepen your connection to the natural world. Every magical step you take will bring you closer to uncovering your full witch's power, ultimate wellness, and authentic self.

Magical Holistic You: Body, Mind, Spirit

Your holistic self is made up of three elements: body, mind, and spirit.

- **The body**, your physical self, is composed of tissues, cells, organs, and complex systems allowing you to move and breathe.

- **The mind**, your mental self, is the essence of who you are, where thoughts, intellect, emotions, and imagination manifest.

- **The spirit**, your spiritual self, is an energetic realm where you're able to access a deeper understanding, awareness, and inner wisdom of yourself and the universe.

These elements create a harmonious triangle capable of bringing the body into a balanced state. It is integral to maintain this balance through exercise for the body, regular stimulation for the mind, nurturing your magical practice for the spirit, and proper nutrition for all three. When your whole self is aligned and thriving, it's easier for your body to maintain this inner balance; the magical energy you put into each act will help get you there.

Taking steps to consciously integrate parts of your magical practice into your daily wellness rituals will help amplify the relationships among mind, body, spirit, and your magic. The more solid these connections, the more balanced you will be. There are many practical things a witch can do each day to help achieve this. For example, you can recite a spell while cooking a healthy meal, utilize the magic of herbs in a healing spell, perform a grounding ritual, or awake each day and give thanks to nature. These daily actions may seem simple, but they will enable you to reach new heights in your wellness and witchcraft practice.

Connecting to your inner magic is another important step toward creating this harmonious triangle of balance. The following ritual is one way to begin building this relationship. By connecting to your inner magic, you can start strengthening the ties among the three pillars of body, mind, and spirit.

Ritual to Connect to Your Inner Magic

Connecting with your inner magic is all about trusting and truly seeing yourself. To know yourself—from the darkest parts to the brightest—is to be present and honestly connected. Learning to tune in to this part of yourself is an excellent first step in your wellness journey. Come back to this ritual whenever you feel this connection needs strengthening. The more you perform this ritual, the easier it will become to access this part of yourself on a regular basis.

You may wish to ground and center yourself before beginning this ritual. (See Chapter 5 for simple grounding and centering rituals.)

Materials to Gather

- Yourself (other items are optional)
- 1 blue candle for spiritual awareness and intuition
- 2 drops patchouli essential oil (properly diluted) for personal growth
- 1 labradorite stone for self-discovery and transformation
- 1 hematite stone for grounding and calm

Steps to Take

1. Find a quiet place where you can relax and sit comfortably.

2. Light your candle. Anoint each wrist with a drop of patchouli oil.

3. Take one stone in each hand and close your eyes. Release any thoughts or feelings from the outside world.

4. Focus first on your physical self. Feel the energy in your body from your toes all the way to the top of your head. Become aware of how you're feeling in this moment.

5. Take a large inhale, exhale, and let your body relax.

6. Visualize yourself sitting cross-legged on a vast crystal floor, the blue sky above and the sunshine glittering down on you. In the center of you emanates a bright white light. All around there are rainbow prisms reflecting off the floor from the sunlight. These rainbow prisms are reflecting into your center light, each one feeding you something different: intuition, inner wisdom, calm, balance, resiliency, love, everything that

makes up your true self. Think on these prisms. What are they reflecting into you? Each reflection is a part of your true self that makes up your inner magic and light. As the rainbows help bring each part of you to light, imagine they are cultivating as a collective whole inside your center. This is where your true self and inner magic live. Hold on to these prisms and focus on the balance and peace they bring to your whole self.

7. Stay in this visualization for at least 5 minutes. Use your intuition to trust when the exercise feels complete. You should feel centered and as light as air.

8. Before finishing, recite the following:

Inner magic, guide me strong,
inner light where I belong.
Free me from thy ego self, and
let me see things clear.
My truest self fully formed,
allowing me to transform.
For now, I can fully see, as my
will so mote it be.

9. Take a few deep breaths, curve your lips into a smile, and open your eyes. You may now extinguish your candle or let it burn down if safe to do so.

Making Magical Wellness a Habit

Habits are behaviors that you partake in so often they become sub-conscious actions, things you automatically do in your daily routine, such as brushing your teeth, having your morning coffee, pulling your daily tarot card, or choosing which crystals you are going to wear each day. Your habits can become so set in your life that it can be challenging to make changes.

One of your major goals in crafting your magical wellness journey is to embrace healthy habits and release the ones that are not serving your holistic self. Become more in tune with your daily routine and ask yourself: Does this action serve me well? Will this action benefit me and my magic? If the answer is no, then that is probably a habit you will want to let go of.

While it's simple to write a schedule or list of angelic (virtuous and good intentioned) goals for yourself, sticking to them requires dedication and mindfulness on your part. Thinking of this new lifestyle as part of your witchcraft practice can help with this. Switching your frame of mind and thinking of your habits as ways to foster not only your wellness but your magic as well will help make it easier to develop healthy habits moving forward. Following are some things to keep in your mind as you embark on this magical new journey.

1. **Keep focus on the magical elements of your new routines.**
Looking at conquering your health goals with the help of magical means will give you a new view of wellness and provide you fresh ways to add magic into your daily life. In fact, the very act of incorporating your magical practice (something that gets you excited) into your wellness practice (something that initially may not provide the same level of enthusiasm) will give you an extra dose of motivation to get moving in a positive direction.

2. **Create a wellness path that you look forward to.** If you plan to go for a run each morning at 6 a.m. and start growing potent powerful witch herbs at home, but you hate running and don't really have the means to grow anything, then you probably aren't going to have much luck sticking with your plan no matter how much magic you weave in. Make your goals realistic and tailored to your personal likes, situation, and witchcraft inclinations. Don't set yourself up for failure by setting the bar too high right away.

3. **Make sure your reasons for starting this journey are your own.** Your reasons should be ones you decide for yourself without outside influences. If you're not truly doing these things for you, it will be much harder to stick to this new lifestyle.

4. **Always consider new ways to weave magic into your wellness.** Instead of simply making a cup of tea, brew a magical potion that will help strengthen you. Instead of just going through the motions of a workout, ground yourself and make that connection with the earth or wear crystals to enhance performance. The more you incorporate your magical energy into your wellness, the easier it will become to do so regularly.

5. **Have patience with yourself and be kind.** Tiny changes done consistently over time add up to remarkable results. And remember, you are a magical star in this universe and deserve to feel your best.

Planning Your Magical Wellness Journey

When starting something new or making changes to something old, whether to your mundane or magical life, it's always wise to have a plan to direct you from where you are to where you want to be. Take some time and think about the different aspects of your wellness and current magical practice. What changes could be made to put you on the road toward your optimal self? Once you figure out your strengths, weaknesses, and ultimate goals, you'll be better equipped to plan the practical and magical elements of your journey.

Try not to rush this planning process. Consider turning it into a ritual for yourself by choosing a quiet space, lighting a candle or incense, or completing a meditation to help find focus and get your magical energies flowing. Whatever method you choose, consider your answers to the following questions carefully:

1. What are your top three wellness goals and how can your magic relate to them?

2. What aspect of yourself (physical, mental, or spiritual) needs the most work?

3. Are there any physical symptoms you suffer from that you'd like to alleviate or any specific body systems that need strengthening? What magical tools may help here?

4. What do you consider to be the strongest parts of yourself based on how you feel each day?

5. Are there any mental blocks you succumb to that you would like to break through?

6. How would you rate your daily energy level? And how does your energy level affect your ability to practice magic?

7. Do you have any undesirable habits you would like to banish?

8. Do you already have wellness rituals that make you happy?

9. If you've tried new healthy routines in the past and failed, what do you think went wrong?

10. What's your favorite part of your magical practice?

11. What are your favorite magical tools to work with?

12. What do you think has been holding you back from reaching your wellness goals?

Once you have clear answers to these questions, it's helpful to record them. This way you can refer back to them and see how far you've come and how things have changed as you've progressed on your path. Your answers could even become an entry in your wellness journal or a page in your grimoire.

Starting a Wellness Journal or Grimoire

There are two types of personal books that many witches hold close to their heart: their journal and their grimoire. Keeping these types of texts is great practice for the witch who enjoys documenting their craft and working their thoughts out through the written word. They can also be helpful for your wellness journey and recording ways you are incorporating your witchcraft practice into your health goals. Let's elaborate on what distinguishes one from the other:

- **Journal:** This is a place where you can record your thoughts, experiences, secrets, and biggest dreams. This type of writing is incredibly therapeutic and helps strengthen the connection to your true self. There are journal prompts included at the end of Chapters 3, 4, and 5 to provide some inspiration for getting started.

- **Grimoire:** This is a book you can keep that is a detailed recording of your magical practice—a place to hold all the magical knowledge you've acquired. In it, you can document information on the Wheel of the Year, properties of herbs and oils, details about deities, or divination experiences. Grimoires are personal to every witch, and what's included is limited only by your practice and areas of interest. If you already have a grimoire, creating a section for magical wellness would be a valuable addition.

It's extremely beneficial to have one, or both, of these texts dedicated to your wellness path. There is so much information you can include that will help keep you on track and connected to your new habits and rituals. Following are some possible content ideas for inspiration. Choose some or all of them to keep track of on your wellness journey. Remember that your magical wellness path is uniquely yours. Some of these ideas may not be right for you, and that's fine. Trust your intuition on what to record, and have fun with it.

- How you feel each day mentally, physically, and spiritually
- What you did today that was beneficial to your holistic wellness
- Daily exercise
- Weekly wellness schedule
- Morning and evening wellness rituals
- Sleep routine
- Daily meals
- Daily macros and/or calories (if you choose to track them)
- Any supplements you're taking and their benefits
- Tea blends you use for specific magical wellness purposes
- Spells and rituals for wellness
- Vitamins or minerals you want to highlight in your daily food intake
- Magical healthy recipes
- Tarot spreads or divination practices relating to your wellness
- Meditations
- Crystals you use for healing and wellness purposes
- Energy center healing practices
- Ways to create space at home where your witchcraft and wellness can work as one

Tools for Magical Wellness

While the most important ingredient in any ritual is your own energy, spirit, and intention, many witches will choose to have some additional tools in their witchcraft arsenal. Working with certain elements in spells and rituals can add a level of power to your workings, creating more desirable results.

Whether or not you choose to work with these items is entirely your decision, and you're not obligated to run out and buy everything mentioned here. This section is meant to give a short overview and provide inspiration for some commonly used elements. Take the following information and tailor your toolbox to meet your own needs.

Herbs

Herbs are generally considered a must-have for any person following a nature-based spiritual path. They're powerful elements that lend themselves to magical and practical healing extremely effectively. If you choose to add one additional tool to your practice, let it be herbs!

That being said, it's incredibly important to know your herbs, use caution, and take care when working with them. Research the source and quality of each of your chosen herbs well, and start slowly (see the chart on the next page).

Crystals

Working with crystals is a staple for many witches. Crystal healing, which has been around for centuries, is an alternative medicine technique based on energy. Crystals take thousands of years to take shape in the earth, and each one carries its own vibrations based on the environment it was formed in. There are many ways to utilize crystals in your magical wellness journey, such as using them in meditation, wearing them as jewelry, placing them strategically around your home, or using them in spell jars and sachets. It is worthwhile to have a few of these in your magical toolbox as their benefits are plentiful (see chart later in this chapter).

Herb	Magical Properties
Basil	Fertility, protection, spiritual growth, strength, optimism, hope, money, cleansing, love, abundance, exorcism
Chamomile	Harmony, prosperity, calm, uplifting, protection, money, sleep, love, purification, meditation, balance, cleansing
Hibiscus	Love, divination, dreams, creativity, passion, healing
Lavender	Happiness, love, relaxation, cleansing, protection, balance, peace, longevity, positive dreams, clairvoyance, purification, calm
Lemon Balm	Love, happiness, purification, healing, renewal, success, calm, fertility, confidence, prosperity
Nettle	Happiness, love, strength, cleansing, protection, balance, peace, longevity, hex breaking
Peppermint	Love, happiness, purity, healing, renewal, success, fertility, energy, divination, money, prosperity, travel, health
Rosemary	Strength, protection, memory, healing, love, purification, intellect, sleep, youthfulness, clarity
Thyme	Courage, ambition, protection, clairvoyance, healing, health, purity, honor ancestors
Valerian	Love, harmony, sleep, purification, protection, astral projection
Yarrow	Happiness, love, divination, courage, balance, peace, longevity, cleansing, protection, psychic abilities, calm

Wellness Properties
Contains antioxidants, may lower blood sugar, mental clarity, alleviates stress, anti-inflammatory, skin health, liver detox
Eases anxiety, aids digestion, wound healing, combats eczema, relieves headaches, encourages sleep, anti-inflammatory
Contains antioxidants, may lower blood pressure, liver health, weight loss, high in polyphenols
Eases anxiety, pain relief, wound healing, combats eczema, induces sleep, eases headaches, relaxes the nervous system, antibacterial
Eases anxiety, aids digestion, fights coughs/colds/cold sores, encourages sleep, boosts brain function, eases nausea
Body detoxification, aids skin conditions, fights acne, combats anemia, contains antioxidants, improves heart health, stimulates lactation, improves allergies
Eases anxiety, aids digestion, boosts energy, improves sleep, fights colds/flus, promotes alertness, enhances cognitive function, relieves headaches
Improves alertness, improves circulation, eases headaches, aids digestion, combats colds/flus, boosts mood, anti-inflammatory
Combats colds/flus, may reduce blood pressure, relaxes muscles, aids digestion, boosts immunity, elevates mood, antimicrobial
Improves sleep, calms nervous system, eases anxiety, relieves muscle pain
Aids digestion, wound healing, balances female reproductive system, fights colds/flus, strengthens blood vessels

Crystal	Magical Properties
Amethyst	Happiness, wisdom, calm, clairvoyance, love, new beginnings, positivity, healing, protection, spirit connection, cleansing, dreams, relaxation
Black Tourmaline	Creativity, grounding, cleansing, strength, protection, healing, positivity, banishing
Carnelian	Confidence, energy, strength, manifestation, happiness, luck, motivation, positivity
Citrine	Inspiration, joy, abundance, optimism, strength, cleansing, confidence, success, intuition
Clear Quartz	Happiness, psychic abilities, cleansing, healing, awareness, balance, optimism, clarity, protection, positivity, meditation
Hematite	Opportunity, balance, self-esteem, banishing, manifestation, strength, calm, grounding, spirit connection
Labradorite	Self-discovery, intuition, creativity, nature, protection, psychic abilities, transformation, awareness, raises vibrations
Lapis Lazuli	Courage, wisdom, insight, balance, intuition, confidence, dreams, truth, spirituality, clarity, air connection
Moonstone	Joy, healing, calm, creativity, harmony, insight, fertility, rebirth, love, dreams, luck, clairvoyance
Peridot	Abundance, prosperity, love, transformation, nature, healing, power, wealth, money
Rose Quartz	Love, joy, creativity, cleansing, healing, balance, fertility, self-esteem, relationships, creativity
Tiger's Eye	Prosperity, money, luck, strength, creativity, focus, protection, intuition, balance, grounding, appreciation, motivation

Wellness Properties
Benefits endocrine system, battles insomnia, pain relief, eases stress, strengthens immune system, benefits skin, relaxes nervous system
Uplifts mood, eases stress, increases energy, protects against EMFs, strengthens immune system
Stimulates metabolism, increases circulation, improves focus, improves absorption of vitamins/minerals, eases back pain
Uplifts mood, aids digestion, improves circulation, balances hormones, energizes, improves focus
Stimulates immune system, improves concentration, boosts metabolism, helps with full-body detox, works as a master healer by bringing balance to the body
Promotes concentration, helps overcome addictions, eases anxiety, fights insomnia, regulates the blood
May lower blood pressure, regulates metabolism, balances hormones, improves circulation, releases anxiety, aids in mental clarity
Combats insomnia, boosts immune system, may lower blood pressure, strengthens thyroid, relaxes nervous system, pain relief
Balances hormones, aids digestion, eases PMS, benefits female reproductive system, eases insomnia
Reduces anxiety, heals tissues, benefits skin, benefits metabolism, improves heart health, combats depression
Boosts brain function, benefits skin, stimulates circulatory system, beneficial to the adrenal glands and female reproductive system
Eases anxiety, healing for eyes and throat, boosts mood, benefits endocrine system, balances hormones

Essential Oil	Magical Properties
Cinnamon	Love, prosperity, strength, success, luck, protection, healing, money, abundance
Clary Sage	Protection, health, longevity, purification, grounding, confidence, wisdom, calm, clairvoyance
Eucalyptus	Healing, purification, protection, growth, banishing
Lemongrass	Love, balance, positivity, psychic awareness, cleansing
Neroli	Happiness, peace, money, relaxation, success, joy, calm
Patchouli	Fertility, personal growth, money, love, passion, success, manifestation, protection, grounding, beauty
Pine	Success, strength, new beginnings, cleansing, banishing, fertility
Sandalwood	Protection, healing, peace, abundance, divination, calm, clarity, banishing, purification
Sweet Orange	Prosperity, luck, love, success, joy, divination, clarity, peace, calm, positivity, protection, happiness
Tea Tree	Peace, strength, protection, cleansing
Vetiver	Grounding, protection, money, love, positivity, luck, breaking hexes, optimism
Ylang-Ylang	Confidence, harmony, happiness, sexuality, calm

Wellness Properties
Eases headaches, antibacterial, treats cuts and bruises, improves circulation, pain relief, aids digestion, may lower blood pressure
Aids digestion, reduces stress, elevates mood, anti-inflammatory, combats menopause symptoms, improves circulation, may reduce blood pressure
Wound healing, eases headaches, combats sinus and lung congestion, pain relief, antibacterial, natural cleanser
Aids digestion, relieves pain, relaxes nervous system, eases headaches, improves mood, promotes alertness, antiseptic properties, natural cleanser
Relaxes the nervous system, improves circulation, eases muscle cramping, encourages sleep, benefits skin, may reduce blood pressure
Fights colds, benefits skin, eases anxiety, relieves headaches, anti-inflammatory
Decreases allergies, relieves muscle pain, boosts mood, promotes mental focus, anti-inflammatory, contains antioxidants, air purifying, energizing
Relaxes the nervous system, improves sleep, combats depression, anti-inflammatory, relieves coughs and sore throats, relieves nausea, calms nervous system, benefits skin
Relaxes the nervous system, eases anxiety, natural cleanser
Wound healing, antibacterial, stimulates immune system, eases skin conditions, fights colds/flus, fights candida, natural cleanser
Fights infection, encourages sleep, skin regeneration, eases anxiety, relieves aches/pains
Relaxes the nervous system, eases anxiety, improves circulation, eases muscle spasms, combats depression, may lower blood pressure, hair health

Essential Oils

Essential oils are naturally occurring aromatic compounds found in the various parts of plants. These oils are made available through a process of distillation, allowing them to retain characteristics from their plant of origin. They are beneficial additions to your witch's cabinet and have a plethora of magical and practical uses you can tap in to (see the chart on the previous page).

Essential Oil Safety

A section on essential oils wouldn't be complete without some safety protocols. Essential oils are very concentrated, and precautions should always be used when working with them.

- Always do a patch test on your skin before using new oils.

- Always dilute with a neutral carrier oil, such as grape-seed, jojoba, coconut, or sweet almond, before applying to the skin. Six to eighteen drops of essential oil per 1-ounce bottle is a safe range. Begin with less and adjust to your preference.

- Never put essential oils directly on open wounds.

- Never ingest essential oils unless properly instructed by a professional. They can be toxic.

- Not all essential oils are suitable for children or pets. Please do your research before giving to each of these vulnerable groups (or using them in their vicinity).

- Some essential oils should be avoided during pregnancy.

- Always read cautions and be knowledgeable about each essential oil you are thinking of working with.

- Essential oils are best stored in dark glass bottles.

- Essential oils will keep at least two years with proper storage. To obtain the longest shelf life, store your essential oils in dark glass bottles away from heat and sunlight. You will know your oil has gone off if there is a noticeable change in the smell, color, consistency, or opaque-ness. And be sure to always check for expiration dates on the packaging.

Candles

Candles are another quintessential tool that witches work with. Candles enable you to incorporate the powerful fire element into your spells and rituals. You can take your candle magic a step further by choosing candles in colors that match your intention; scribing them with symbols, runes, or sigils; and dressing them with appropriate herbs and oils. When purchasing candles, it is best to try and stay away from paraffin wax candles, opting instead for natural materials such as soy or beeswax. These materials provide you a better connection with the earth and will not release harmful toxins into the air. Here are some color associations you can use when choosing candles, as well as ribbons and other elements for your spells and rituals.

- **White:** purification, strength, cleansing, clarity, spirit connection, blessings, renewal

- **Pink:** friendship, love, romance, tranquility, beauty, emotional healing, happiness, self-esteem, youth

- **Purple:** power enhancement, healing, ambition, divination, reversing curses, wisdom, spirituality, purpose, higher self

- **Red:** health, protection, vitality, sexuality, passion, strength, courage, represents fire

- **Orange:** encouragement, concentration, vitality, intellect, creativity, attraction, good luck

- **Yellow:** intelligence, charm, confidence, joy, travel, clairvoyance, represents air, optimism

- **Blue:** dreams, calm, sleep protection, spiritual awareness, peace, intuition, insight, represents water, tranquility, serenity, healing, patience, communication

- **Green:** fertility, success, prosperity, luck, harmony, healing, connection to nature, balance, wealth, abundance, money

- **Silver:** moon representation, confidence, intuition, gratitude, dreams, psychic abilities, blessings

- **Gold:** sun representation, wealth, generosity, overcoming addiction, abundance, positivity, money

- **Brown:** stability, animals and pets, friendships, gardening, house blessing, represents earth

- **Black:** loss, sadness, releasing negativity, protection, banishing, power

Practical Tools

Here are some additional tools you may wish to have while working through this book's activities and are by no means mandatory. This list is meant to outline items specific to what this book recommends, not to list every tool that some witches typically have.

- Mortar and pestle
- Various incense
- Double boiler
- Glass jars/bottles of different sizes
- 4–12-ounce spray bottles (glass if possible)
- 1-ounce dark glass dropper bottles
- Small cloth pouches in different colors

- Cauldron
- Measuring spoons
- Stainless steel funnels
- Method to diffuse essential oils (see Chapter 2)
- Notebook or binder
- Special writing utensils
- Small decorative boxes

Your witch's tool kit, like your magical wellness path, will be unique to you. There are multiple different herbs, oils, crystals, or colors that can be used with equal effectiveness to achieve the same goals. Choose the things that call to you and leave the ones that don't. The items you decide to add into your practice will evolve with your journey and as you acquire new knowledge and experience. Experiment with different elements, explore new magical techniques, and enjoy the process of discovery.

CHAPTER TWO

Creating a Magical Environment That Fosters Wellness

Creating a magical environment where you can nurture your witchcraft practice, as well as feel safe, secure, and happy, plays a critical role in your magical wellness journey. The witch's home is a sanctuary, a sacred space, and a place where the most powerful magic can take shape.

Your home should feed your magical self and, in turn, your magic should feed your home. The stronger these connections, the more content you will feel in other areas of your life. You want your space to bring joy and feel light and airy all while making you, and others, feel magical just by being in it. There are many ways to incorporate magical energy into the home, including cleaning techniques, protection rituals and positivity spells, and even your decor.

This chapter will explore setting up your space to encourage wellness and magic, benefits of natural and sustainable living, and how to magically cleanse and protect the home, as well as recipes for cleansers, herb sachets, and oil blends. Through the suggestions and activities in this chapter, your space will undergo a transformation that will have a positive effect on the energies within your home and yourself.

Your home is the place where you spend most of your time and where a lot, or possibly all, of your magical work is done. If you want to have a strong and abundant witchcraft practice, you will need to create an environment with energies to support that. A chaotic home will equal a chaotic body, mind, and spirit, making it difficult to perform spell work that is fruitful and stays on track with your wellness goals. But if your home has lovely, free-flowing energy, the same will be encouraged within yourself, manifesting to reveal a healthier, more dynamic, and balanced witch.

Houses have their own energy that they acquire over the years from the land and all of those who have passed their threshold. Connecting with the inherent energies of your home and taking time to learn about and connect with the land on which your dwelling sits can create powerful relationships among yourself, the land, and your home. Spend time learning the land's history, and become familiar with the plants, trees, and wildlife that live around you. Be grateful and honor the energies of this magical piece of earth where you have made a home.

Set up your space in a manner that is pleasing to you and allows a balanced flow of energy. Your home should project your personality, speak to you, and bring a smile to your lips. So how do you take control of your space and begin to align it with your unique magical energy? Try the following detox ritual for help.

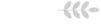

Magical Detox Ritual

In order to flourish, your magic requires a cleansed space where energies flow naturally. The process of detoxing will help to create this fluidity within your home. The act of releasing conventional products from your life will assist in clearing away blockages, creating a space where your magic and holistic self can thrive. This ritual will solidify these intentions and help you begin letting go of the toxic items in your household.

Materials to Gather

- 1 stick eucalyptus incense for purification and growth
- Paper and a pen
- Trowel or another tool for digging
- Small pot with soil, or a spot outside where you can dig a hole

Steps to Take

1. Cleanse, ground, and center as needed.

2. Relax and ease your mind. For this ritual, you want to focus on changing things in your home that will help eliminate toxins from the environment. What items will it be beneficial for you to let go of?

3. Sit comfortably and light your incense. Allow yourself to embrace the cleansing energy it holds. Open yourself up to this new venture of personal growth.

4. Take your paper and pen and make a list of everything you would like to detox from your home. Maybe it's conventional cleaning products, processed foods, paraffin candles, or the standard facial makeup you've gotten used to. Whatever it may be, put it on the list. Once your list is complete, recite the following:

> *Toxicity, you have no place,*
> *in my life or in my space.*
> *I cleanse you from my house and home,*
> *this is my will; it's set in stone.*

5. Now take the list and tear it up. Gather the pieces of paper, dig a hole in your soil, and then bury the pieces. This action symbolizes these things making an exit from your home and life.

6. Alternatively, if you are able to do so safely, you can burn the list in your cauldron or a firesafe dish instead. The symbolism will remain the same.

Sustainable living is caring for the earth in hands-on ways. It means taking into consideration how your daily actions will impact the environment around you. When you choose to make your own household cleaners, shop from local farmers, or purchase soy candles for your magical practice, these are sustainable choices. Making these decisions creates stronger connections among yourself, the earth, and your magic. The following ritual will allow you to express gratitude to the earth and make the commitment to embrace a more sustainable lifestyle.

Gratitude Ritual to Mother Earth

Giving thanks and respecting Mother Earth is an essential aspect of a witch's life. Showing gratitude and connecting with nature will relieve stress, increase feelings of positivity, manifest more solid spell work, and provide a sense of purpose. The energies of the earth will become more accessible in your magical workings as you establish a relationship with the spirits of nature. These are key elements to achieving an overall state of total wellness. When you commit to healing the earth, you are also committing to healing yourself.

Materials to Gather

- Outdoor space (required, so wait for a nice day)
- Paper and pen (optional)

Steps to Take

1. Take a walk around your neighborhood. Regardless of whether your neighborhood is in a city or beside a sprawling forest, take this walk with all your senses wide open. Release anything else from your mind.

2. While you're walking, take in the natural elements that surround you—maybe there is a tree-lined

street, a flowing river, or gardens filled with beautiful greenery and blossoms. Whatever parts of nature surround you, really open your eyes and appreciate the natural magic of it all. Breathe in the intoxicating smells deeply and hear the sounds all around you. Becoming more aware of the natural beauty will open new channels in your magical practice. Take at least 15 minutes for this step.

3. Choose a place close to your home that you feel comfortable in for the second part of this ritual, where you will affirm your new commitment to the earth. It could be in a park, a grassy field, or your own yard.

4. Once you have your location, sit comfortably, feel the earth beneath you, take off your shoes, and feel the ground and grass beneath your feet. Settle yourself and take a few deep breaths while focusing on the beauty that surrounds you in nature each day.

5. If your surroundings allow it, recite the following aloud. This also can be said silently in your mind if that is more comfortable for you.

I commit to healing you, our Mother Earth.
I commit to sustainable habits and routines.
My gratitude is great and I will express it each day.
You will be honored within my house, my home, myself.
This is my commitment to you.
From this day forward, I shall see it through.

6. Close your eyes and give a final thanks to the earth.

7. These final two steps are optional once you are back at home. Get a paper and pen and make a list of the first steps you will take on your path to more sustainable living. What changes might you be able to make today, tomorrow, or next week? Place your list on your refrigerator or somewhere you will see it regularly as a reminder of this new promise.

8. Lastly, make a list of any habits you currently have that do not honor nature, and burn the list in your cauldron or a firesafe dish to symbolize your letting them go.

Welcoming nature into your household is an exceedingly healthy practice. Having plants in the home can lower stress, improve mood, encourage productivity, and provide some much-needed enchanting earth energy within your space. Creating an environment that perks you up, promotes relaxation, and feeds your magical spirit is essential, which makes adopting a plant or two an easy decision. Having plants—or even just one—will provide many benefits to your home, magic, and overall wellness.

Plant Blessing Ritual

Plants are living organisms filled with their own energies that can breathe new life and happiness into your space. Every witch should have at least one plant friend to care for. It is good to welcome and bless a new plant that has found a home with you. This simple ritual is filled with love and positivity to help you foster a strong bond with your new plant from day one.

Materials to Gather

- Your new plant
- 1 stick peppermint incense for love, healing, and good health
- 1 moss agate stone for vitality and connection to nature

Steps to Take

1. Cleanse, ground, and center as needed.

2. Once your plant is placed in its new home, set your incense nearby and light it.

3. Take a moment to appreciate your new plant. Take in its leaves, branches, and scents. Appreciate the beauty that nature has allowed you to enjoy inside your home. Visualize it growing strong and thriving. Spend at least 5 minutes with this step.

4. Recite the following:

Beauty so green and filled with life, I send to you love and light.
Energy to grow full and strong, lush and thriving all day long.

5. Place your agate inside the plant's pot and say: "May this moss agate bring you vitality and long life."

6. Give thanks to your plant and to Mother Nature for this wonderful gift. You may let the incense burn down fully if you wish.

Excess items in a space block energy, leaving it to become heavy, stagnant, and stuffy. This type of energy is not beneficial to your well-being or magical practice. Once you begin to declutter your space, it will feel as though a weight has been lifted from your shoulders. You will be making space for the energies within your home to flow freely. The air will feel lighter, brighter, and more conducive to the magical work that you do. More space within the home equals more space within your mind. This shift will revitalize your energy, allowing more room for things that feed you, like your witchcraft practice.

Ritual for Letting Go of Material Possessions

When your home is clear of unnecessary possessions, the energy will become more luminous, with the ability to flow unburdened. This ritual will help you make peace with letting go, provide that little push to get started, and bring you one step closer to wellness and your ideal witch's home.

Materials to Gather

- 1 white candle for purification, clarity, and strength
- 1 stick lemon balm incense for renewal, success, and happiness
- Piece of paper and a pen
- Glass of drinking water for cleansing, healing, and flexibility

Steps to Take

1. Cleanse, ground, and center as needed.

2. Find a quiet space where you won't be disturbed. This can be at your altar or another sacred space in your home where you feel relaxed.

3. Sit comfortably, then light your candle and incense.

4. Take three deep breaths to slow your heart rate and promote calm in the body. Allow feelings of gratitude, confidence, and control to fill your mind.

5. Close your eyes and take a moment to visualize what you would like your most perfect witch's dwelling to look like. Visualize your space as being clean, uncluttered, and overflowing with magical energy. Simply picturing your space in this ideal state will promote feelings of happiness and determination to turn it into reality. Think about how you will feel coming home to a space that is beautiful, organized, and uplifting—an ideal place to perform your spells and rituals. Imagine how well your magic will flow when the energies are unburdened by material things. Envision a beautiful, sparkling white glitter dust flowing freely in and around the space. Spend a few moments in this visualization.

6. Retrieve your paper and pen and write three empowering affirmations that align with your decluttering goals, such as the following:

I release what no longer serves.
I am motivated, strong, and focused.
A clean and organized home is within my control.

7. Once you have written down your affirmations, set the paper in front of you and recite the following:

I release the things I no longer need.
Let the energy in this space be freed.
Clean, clear, and filled with light.
Energy focused, strong, and bright.
As my will, it shall be done.

8. Open your eyes and drink the glass of water. Embracing the vital water element brings forth powerful healing, cleansing, and flexible energies, as well as a sense of freedom. Water ebbs, flows, and moves with the tides. Allow yourself to invoke the ability to have fluid energies that easily adapt throughout this process. While you drink, you may focus on your task ahead. Think about what room or element in your home you will start with and focus on how you will feel once you bring your earlier visualization into reality.

9. Once you have finished your water, simply say, "I am thankful; I am grateful; I am blessed for all that I have and am ready to let things go." This work is now complete. You may extinguish your candle and incense or allow them to burn down fully if safe to do so.

Decluttering is a great opportunity to donate to charities and help others. Share the wealth. Don't simply throw everything into the trash. That is not helpful to your fellow humans or the environment. Make sure you put aside items and clothing in good condition that can be given to those in need. Consider performing an easy blessing ritual on these items before they go to their new owners. You may simply place your hand over the item and state, "May this item be blessed for its journey to come," or run an incense stick that encourages hope and positivity, such as basil, over the item.

Physical and energetic cleansing are imperative to your magical wellness journey, the health of your home, and your witchcraft practice as a whole. Before tackling energetic cleansing by clearing out negative and stagnant energies from your home, it's important to physically clean your space. The act of cleaning and moving things shifts energies and releases dust and particles into the air, so it's good sense to complete this task first. So how do you magically cleanse your home? To magically cleanse is simply weaving your own magical ingredients, spells, and intentions into your physical cleaning tasks. A shining example of everyday witchcraft.

The amount of essential oils you use for each of these recipes can vary depending on your preference and whether you like it more or less scented. Just make sure to use at least a few drops so that you get the benefits of their natural cleansing and magical properties.

Here are some magical cleaning tips that will enable you to add specific energies and intentions throughout the process.

Magical Cleaning Techniques

- Use floral waters in your cleansing mixtures, such as lavender for happiness or chamomile for balance.

- Use water that you have charged by the moon or sun with specific intentions.

- Always sweep and mop toward the exit of the room. This signifies moving negativity and unwanted energies out of the space.

- Have a separate broom for when you are doing purposeful magical cleansings as opposed to when you're simply sweeping up everyday spills: your magical besom, used for ritual purposes, and your everyday broom, used for mundane tasks.

- Use cleansers that you mix yourself; they are another form of magical potions. Be sure to set intentions while you prepare them.

- Utilize visualization while cleaning. Visualize a happy home, a balanced home, a home filled with abundance and light, or whatever matches your intentions at the time.

- Recite chants or spells while you clean that strengthen and make clear your intentions.

- Make a witch's playlist to have on while cleaning or mixing your cleansers. Music that moves you can really get those magical energies flowing and inspired.

There are several easy ways to energetically cleanse your space prior to performing magical work as suggested throughout these rituals. You may use incense, such as lavender, rosemary, or lemon balm; a cleansing mist (see recipe provided in this chapter), with sound from bells or cymbals; or by placing cleansing crystals, such as clear quartz or citrine, in your space.

All-Purpose Cleaner for Purifying Your Space

Conventional cleaning products are filled with chemicals that can be readily absorbed into the body, contributing to physical and magical blockages within yourself. Crafting your own is a great skill that allows you to perform some everyday magic, embrace your inner hearth witch, and minimize or avoid certain health problems such as asthma, allergies, and skin conditions.

Magical properties: healing, purification, peace, uplifting energies, protection, strength

Materials to Gather

- 1 cup distilled water
- ½ cup white vinegar
- 2 tablespoons liquid castile soap (such as Dr. Bronner's)
- 10 drops eucalyptus essential oil
- 5 drops lemongrass essential oil
- 5 drops tea tree essential oil
- 12-ounce spray bottle

Steps to Take

1. Cleanse, ground, and center as needed.

2. Simple mixing method: Add all ingredients into a spray bottle, shake it up, et voilà!

3. Adding a dash of magic: As you add each ingredient into your spray bottle, take your time and do so with intention. Visualize that with each spray of this magical mixture, you will be cleansing your space of negativity and welcoming warm, joyful, and prosperous energies in its place.

4. While mixing the ingredients, recite the following three times:

> Cleanse this space and set it free.
> Bring warmth and joy, so mote it be.

5. This cleanser should be stored in a cool, dry space away from direct sunlight. It is also good practice to shake before each use to ensure all ingredients are well mixed as separation will naturally occur.

Bathroom Cleanser for Clarity

This bathroom cleaner will cleanse, fight mold, and bring a sense of peace to the space thanks to the essential oils and alcohol content. **Magical properties:** cleansing, success, clarity, peace, calm, strength, prosperity, joy

Materials to Gather

- 1 cup distilled water
- ⅓ cup rubbing alcohol or vodka
- 2 tablespoons liquid castile soap (such as Dr. Bronner's)
- 10 drops tea tree essential oil
- 5 drops peppermint essential oil
- 5 drops sweet orange essential oil
- 10–12-ounce spray bottle

Steps to Take

1. Prepare in the same manner as the All-Purpose Cleaner for Purifying Your Space (see recipe in this chapter). While mixing, recite the following:

Cleanse this space and set it free.

Bring peace and calm, so mote it be.

2. This cleanser should be stored in a cool, dry space away from direct sunlight. It is also good practice to shake before each use to ensure all ingredients are well mixed as separation will naturally occur.

Energized Glass Cleaner

This simple, yet effective, glass cleaner has only a few ingredients. It is imbued with energies of love, beauty, and confidence—things you should always feel when looking into a mirror and energies that a well-balanced home should certainly contain.

Magical properties: prosperity, love, beauty, confidence, success

Materials to Gather

- 1 cup distilled water
- ⅓ cup rubbing alcohol
- 3 tablespoons white vinegar
- 1 tablespoon cornstarch
- 10 drops lemon essential oil
- 5 drops grapefruit essential oil
- 10–12-ounce spray bottle

Steps to Take

1. Prepare in the same manner as the All-Purpose Cleaner for Purifying Your Space (see recipe in this chapter). While mixing, recite the following:

Cleanse this space and set it free.
Bring love and beauty, so mote it be.

2. This cleanser should be stored in a cool, dry space away from direct sunlight. It is also good practice to shake before each use to ensure all ingredients are well mixed as separation will naturally occur.

Banishing Floor Wash

Washing the floors is an opportune time for a witch to perform cleansing and banishing magic throughout the home. To use this floor wash, you can either put it into a spray bottle and spray your floors as you go or add the entire mixture into your mop bucket with some additional water. Simply add the mixture to your regular mop bucket and fill remaining space with water as you normally would.

Magical properties: purification, protection, banishing, happiness

Materials to Gather

- 2 cups distilled water
- 1 cup white vinegar
- ½ cup witch hazel
- 10 drops pine essential oil
- 10 drops tea tree essential oil
- 10 drops bergamot essential oil

Steps to Take

1. Prepare in the same manner as the All-Purpose Cleaner for Purifying Your Space (see recipe in this chapter), focusing your energy and setting the intention of cleansing your space and banishing negative energies while you're mixing the ingredients. Recite the following while mixing to set this intention:

> *Cleanse and banish negativity. Transform this space, so mote it be.*

2. This cleanser should be stored in a cool, dry space away from direct sunlight. It is also good practice to shake before each use to ensure all ingredients are well mixed as separation will naturally occur.

Ritual Floor Cleansing to Banish Negativity

This floor cleansing is an ideal ritual for cleansing as it simultaneously cleans your space both physically and energetically. You may perform this banishing ritual once per season or whenever you feel the space needs a reset.

Steps to Take

1. Cleanse, ground, and center as needed.

2. Prepare the Banishing Floor Wash (see recipe in this chapter). Remember to set your intentions and visualize your desired outcome while you do this.

3. Prior to beginning to mop, sit comfortably in the center of your most frequented room, breathe deep, and calm your mind, then recite the following:

> I banish thee from within
> these walls,
> Mother goddess, hear my call.
> Negativity, I set you free.
> As my will, so mote it be.

4. Now you may begin to mop. Start at the back of your home and move throughout each space until you reach your front entrance. With every swish of your mop, imagine the negative energies becoming little gray water droplets that lift up and away, dissipating out into the ether. Hold this visualization throughout the process.

5. Once you have finished going through each room, sit in a comfortable position in the same room you started mopping in. However, now you are in your freshly cleansed space and acknowledging that your task is complete. Close your eyes if you wish and recite the following:

> This space is cleansed.
> This space is freed.
> May the energies be bright.
> From morning through night.

6. Open your eyes and give thanks to the energies of your home. Your work is now complete.

Cinnamon Broom Cleansing Ritual

A broom cleansing is a perfect way to clear unwanted energies from your space.

Materials to Gather

- 1 stick lavender incense for purification, happiness, and balance
- Magical besom
- Small amount of cinnamon spice or essential oil for protection, prosperity, love, and luck

Steps to Take

1. Cleanse, ground, and center as needed.

2. Begin in a central room in your home. Clear your mind, focus on the task at hand, and light your incense.

3. Anoint your besom with either your cinnamon spice or oil. Rubbing just a little into the bristles and/or on the handle will do. You do not need much.

4. Move to the back room of your home. This is where you will begin your magical sweeping. When you're sweeping energy from a space, your besom doesn't need to actually touch the floor as you're not sweeping up physical dirt. You may simply brush the air in a sweeping motion.

5. Go through each room of your home pushing the unwanted energies toward the door with your besom. While sweeping, imagine the energies swirling up and away like a cloud of smoke out the door. Focus on feel-good emotions and positivity throughout this process.

6. You will end your sweeping at the front door of your home. When finished, make a point of opening your front door and then closing it firmly. This signifies the energies leaving your space and not being invited back in.

7. Proceed back to the room where you lit your incense. Hold your broom out in front of you horizontally and recite the following to recognize the task you have just completed:

> *The energy within has been reborn.*
> *My home now cleansed, balanced, and free.*
> *This is my will, so mote it be.*

8. Let the incense burn down fully if safe to do so.

Cleansing Simmer Pot

Every witch should have a good simmer pot recipe or two in their magical arsenal. This is a simple and effective cleansing that is great to perform when you feel your space needs some refreshed energy but you don't have time for a long ritual.

Materials to Gather

- Small pot filled with water
- 2 bay leaves for cleansing and purification
- 6 slices lemon for joy
- 1 stick cinnamon for good luck
- 1 tablespoon pure vanilla extract for love

Steps to Take

1. Cleanse, ground, and center as needed.

2. Gather your ingredients and clear your mind. Focus on the intention of clearing out any negativity or unwanted energy from your home. Visualize a home full of calm, joyful, and renewed energies—a fresh start for creating your magical environment.

3. Place your pot filled with water on the stove and turn on your burner to medium-high heat.

4. Add in the ingredients one at a time. While adding in each ingredient, focus on the properties it carries.

5. Once all the ingredients are added, stir the contents with a wooden spoon in a clockwise direction three times to promote positivity and good fortune.

6. Allow the pot to come to a boil. Keep focus on your intentions during this time.

7. Once the mixture is boiling, turn the heat down to low and allow to simmer. Recite the following:

> This home be cleansed; this home be pure.

> Negativity, I let you go; it's time for love and joy to flow.

8. Let the pot simmer for as long as you would like but be sure not to let it boil dry. If you'd like to keep it going, just add more water when it gets low.

It's most effective to repeat this process; simmer pot once a day for 2–3 days. The ingredients are fine to be reboiled, and repeating the process can amplify your spell as a whole. Simply compost your ingredients (if applicable) once your cleansing is complete.

When crafting magical potions that include a stirring action, the direction you choose to stir can impact your results. Generally speaking, if you wish to draw something to yourself or add positivity to the work, stir clockwise, and if your intention is to banish or repel something, stir counterclockwise. If you stir in the wrong direction don't fret, just reiterate your intentions and switch to the correct direction. Feel free to choose for yourself how often and for how long you choose to incorporate this particular practice.

Just like you need to balance energies within yourself, you must also create a balanced and harmonious flow inside your home. Once you've cleansed away undesirable energies from your space, it is wise to perform a balancing spell, home blessing, or both.

This ritual will have you focus on bringing harmony between the spiritual and vibrational energies within your space. While you don't want the energies to be too low, you also don't want them too high as that can be equally draining on you. Performing a home blessing is a wonderful way to even out these energies. It will add positivity to your space while promoting a calm and harmonious atmosphere.

Witch's Home Blessing

For this home blessing, you will focus on creating a space that promotes relaxation, combats anxiety, and lends itself to your magical practice. Before beginning, make sure your home is fully cleansed. If it's not, you will be blessing a space with unbalanced and possibly negative energies. This is counterproductive to your goal of creating a home that lends itself to fostering wellness and amplifying your magical workings.

Materials to Gather

- 1 white jar candle for purification and blessings (this could also be a votive candle on a plate; just make sure it is safe to be carried)
- 1 stick yarrow incense to promote balance, peace, and happiness
- 1 rose quartz stone for balance, love, and healing

Steps to Take

1. Cleanse, ground, and center as needed.

2. Choose a central location in your home and position yourself comfortably with your materials.

3. Place your candle, incense, and crystal into a triangle shape in front of you with the candle as the top point.

4. Take three deep breaths to center yourself and clear your mind. Your thoughts should be focused only on the task at hand.

5. Light your candle and say, "Flame of pure bright light, send blessings to this space."

6. Now light your incense and say, "Sacred yarrow, lend your balancing energies to this space."

7. Sit with your eyes closed and visualize your home being swept through with waves of rainbow light. The rays wash the space in positivity with all of the uplifting colors that the rainbow holds. Imagine yourself in your space living each day with feelings of joy, hopefulness, love, and so much light. Stay in this visualization for a few minutes until you feel it's complete.

8. Stand and carry your candle with you. Now walk through each room of your home and recite the following upon entering each:

This home be blessed with pure rainbow light.
This home be blessed from morning through night.
Balance, peace, and harmony, within this space, so shall it be.

Visualize the rainbow light once again sweeping through each room as you go and then imagine the rainbow light leaving behind an array of twinkling white lights.

9. Once you have gone through each room, return to your starting point and place the candle back at the top of the triangle. Extinguish your candle and say, "And it is done." If safe, allow your incense to burn down fully.

Protecting the home from negative energy, unwanted visitors, and any ill wishes, both psychic and temporal, is crucial to your overall mind frame and emotional state. Feeling safe and secure in your most sacred space is of the utmost importance. Using magical means to enhance this feeling can lessen stress, ease anxiety, and bring a sense of calm and comfort to the home. Think of these workings as magical locks and keys.

You can put up magical protection barriers both outside and inside of the home. Following are some ideas for each:

Magical Protection for Outside the Home

- Place a broom outside your front entrance.

- Hang two brooms of any size crossed above your entrance.

- Sprinkle dried sage, nettle, or dragon's blood resin across your front threshold.

- Bury a pouch of salt under your steps or place the pouch by your entrance to protect from unwanted spirits.

- Place marigolds outside the home.

- Trace a pentacle on your front door with salt water.

- Place protection stones such as amethyst, black tourmaline, or tiger's eye in your garden or by your door.

- Paint your front door black, a protective color.

- Hang bells or wind chimes outside the home.

Magical Protection for Inside the Home

- Use protective essential oils such as cinnamon, eucalyptus, or tea tree when you clean.

- Trace a pentacle or other protective symbols or sigils in key places around your home.

- Have protective elements of oak, cedar, or ebony in your home. This could be full furniture pieces or small things like a candle holder or picture frame.

- Keep a fern inside your home.

- Hang a rope of garlic or onions in your kitchen (not to be used for cooking). Simply compost (if applicable) and replace when necessary.

- Keep a mortar and pestle in your kitchen.

- Utilize herb sachets and crystal pouches throughout your home.

- Recite a protection spell in each room of your home. Consider using the protection room mist from this chapter when it feels called for.

- Have something black in every room to protect and ground the space.

Ritual for Protecting Your Front Entrance

The front entrance is an important area to apply protection to as it is a main point of entry for guests and all sorts of energy. By putting up magical protection, you're deterring anything negative or unsavory from entering. This ritual will be performed just outside your front entrance. If you're in an apartment building, it will be performed on the outside of your apartment's front door, not the main building entrance.

Materials to Gather

- 1–2 drops sweet orange essential oil (properly diluted) for protection, love, and prosperity
- 1 teaspoon dried nettle for protection, happiness, and peace

Steps to Take

1. Cleanse, ground, and center as needed. You may also wish to cast a protective circle around your space prior to beginning (see Chapter 5). Make sure you're feeling calm and relaxed. Leave any negativity from your day at the door, so to speak.

2. Take a long deep breath and place a drop or two of sweet orange oil onto your index finger and gently trace a pentacle on your door. It can be as large or small as you wish. As you do this, recite the following: "Sweet orange oil, protect this space and bathe it in love and light."

3. When you finish stating this, imagine the pentacle illuminating in a bright white light.

4. Take your dried nettle and

sprinkle it across the doorway threshold then recite the following: "Magical nettle, herb of the earth, protect this space from harm." Now visualize that same bright white light illuminating up from your threshold and around the doorframe.

5. Close your eyes and recite the following three times:

> *This home is protected; this home is secure.*
> *Negativity be banned and evil be shunned.*

6. Give thanks for this protective blessing.

Harnessing Fire for Protection

This simple candle ritual will harness the powerful and transformational energy of the fire element and the protective properties of the color black, along with a magical spell to create protection barriers within your home.

Materials to Gather

- 1 black candle for protection and banishing

Steps to Take

1. Cleanse, ground, and center as needed.

2. Choose a quiet place in your home where you will not be disturbed. This can be at your altar or any space where you feel relaxed and balanced.

3. Sit comfortably and light your candle.

4. Take three deep breaths and focus your gaze on the flame. Visualize black sparkles of glitter rising up from the flame and traveling throughout your home. Imagine them traveling the perimeter of each room with special attention to doors, windows, and mirrors, which can all be entryways for unwelcome energy. Stay in this visualization until you see the black glitter circulate through your entire home.

5. Close your eyes and recite the following:

> *Bright burning flame, secure this place*

Shield it from harm in time and space.
Fire element, hear my call.
May your protective energy build a wall.
With this I give my thanks and love.

From the earth below to the sky above.

6. Open your eyes, give thanks to the fire element, and say, "So mote it be."

7. Now extinguish your flame.

Manipulating Energy with a Crystal Grid

A dynamic way to add crystals into your practice is by creating a crystal grid. Crystal grids are a powerful tool for manipulating the energy within a space. With a grid, you are creating shapes with various crystals that work together synergistically to manifest your specific intention. They can be set up for a multitude of purposes such as prosperity, positivity, happiness, or, of course, protection.

Crystal grids are really a piece of magical art, so feel free to get creative with the way you place your crystals. You will need to choose a spot for your grid where it can stay undisturbed and also where you are able to see it each day. The exact number of stones you use is up to you. Here, seven stones are suggested, but you can choose an amount that feels appropriate for you.

Materials to Gather

- 1 stick chamomile incense for cleansing
- 1 clear quartz stone to ward against negativity and encourage positivity (ideally, it should be larger than the rest of the stones you use)
- 2 hematite stones for banishing negativity
- 2 black tourmaline stones for grounding energy
- 2 amethyst stones for protection
- Piece of paper and a pen
- Wand or pointed crystal (optional)

Steps to Take

1. Cleanse, ground, and center as needed.

2. Gather your crystals and choose your space.

3. Place your crystals in the space and do a quick cleansing for both. You want the energy around that space and the stones themselves to

be pure and untainted. Do this by lighting your incense and letting the smoke absorb any energies surrounding the space. Wave the incense around, through the space, and over the crystals until you are satisfied all of them are well cleared.

4. Take your piece of paper and pen and clearly write your intention. For example, write something like: "This crystal grid is created to protect my space from negativity and harm."

5. Fold your paper into three and place it in the center of where your grid will be.

6. Now take your clear quartz and place it in the center of your grid on top of the paper with your intention written on it.

7. Place the other stones in a circle shape around your center stone, alternating the stones as you go. The shape should be symmetrical in nature so that the stones may work together synergistically. Feel free to get creative and add to this basic setup if you feel compelled. You can add as many layers to the grid as you like.

8. Next, state your intention out loud to solidify its nature to the universe. You may say what you wrote on the paper or you can say, "This crystal grid is empowered to protect my space from negativity and harm."

9. Lastly, activate your grid. You may use your wand for this step instead of your hand if you wish. Take your hand and hover it above your center stone. Now imagine a black string moving from one stone to the next as your hand moves around the circle, connecting all the stones. Finish with your hand back above your center stone. Hold this image of the connected stones for a moment and thank the stones and the earth for their service.

10. Leave your grid up for as long as you feel it is serving its purpose.

If you enjoy this process and the concept of crystal grids, you may utilize these steps for any intention you have for yourself simply by switching out the crystals so that they match your intention.

MANIFESTING PROSPERITY IN THE HOME

Ensuring prosperity and abundance in the home can do wonders for your mental health. Working some abundance magic centered around your home can help to assure your bills are paid and there is always food on the table.

Keep in mind that when talking about spells and rituals that concern finances, it is the same as with anything else: You must do the work—yes, your magical work, but also everyday practical work. You can't simply perform a money spell and then the next day expect money to just appear in your bank account. You must still take practical steps. Your magical work is meant to enhance your means and shift energies to work for you, but practical work must still be done.

Manifesting a Prosperous Home

This ritual is about ensuring you will have what you need and will not go without—it will help ensure security, not extravagance. If possible, wait to perform it when the moon is full, which is the moon's most powerful phase and an optimal time to perform prosperity magic. Alternatively, you can perform it on a Thursday evening. Thursday is ruled by Jupiter, which makes it the most influential day to perform prosperity magic.

Materials to Gather

- 1–2 drops cinnamon essential oil (properly diluted) for prosperity and success
- 1 green candle for prosperity and luck

Steps to Take

1. Cleanse, ground, and center as needed.

2. Sit comfortably in your space, place a drop or two of the cinnamon oil on your index finger, and anoint your candle with it. Run your finger up the sides and around the center until you are satisfied. Be sure to use only a small amount of oil.

3. Now light your candle and close your eyes. Visualize your home as having everything it needs. The cupboards are full, the bills all have "paid" stamped on them, and

everything is running smoothly. Feel in your core the emotions this scenario will bring to you: relief, relaxation, peace, joy. Stay in this visualization for at least 5 minutes. Let your mind wander free with the knowledge that everything within the home is secure and well.

4. Once you finish, open your eyes and recite the following:

This home will prosper; this home will bloom,
all needs be met within these rooms.
Sacred flame burning bright, make it so this magical night.

5. Give thanks, say, "So it shall be done," and extinguish your flame.

Drawing Money Into the Home

This spell jar is specifically directed toward manifesting more money in order to ease an area of stress in your life. Perhaps you have some debt you worry about constantly or you want to manifest a raise at your main job so you can quit your second one, or maybe you just really need a vacation but require more funds to pay for it.

Materials to Gather

- 1 tablespoon dried chamomile for money and prosperity
- 1 tablespoon dried basil for money and fertility
- 1 tablespoon dried peppermint for money and renewal
- Mortar and pestle
- Small glass jar with lid
- 3 coins to represent wealth
- 1 peridot stone for money and wealth
- 3 drops patchouli essential oil for growth and success
- 1 green string or ribbon for wealth (long enough to tie around your jar)

Steps to Take

1. Cleanse, ground, and center as needed.

2. Choose your workspace and gather your ingredients. You may wish to perform this ritual in the kitchen or at your altar.

3. Place each of your three herbs into your mortar one at a time. Take

your pestle and begin to blend the herbs together. While you do this, visualize yourself without any money troubles. Imagine a bank account with a nice positive balance, a wallet that is full, and debts that are paid; whatever money issues may be plaguing you, imagine them as no longer being a problem. You have more than enough for your needs. Let the feelings of happiness and relief wash over you. Really manifest them deep in your core, let your lips smile, and relax your shoulders. All is well.

4. Once you finish blending, you will begin adding ingredients into your jar. First, add in the coins and say,

"Money flows to me easily." Then add in your herb blend and say, "My bank account grows each day." Next, add in your crystal and say, "I attract wealth." Lastly, add in your drops of patchouli oil and say: "Money is no longer a source of stress."

5. Place the lid securely on your jar, then take your green string or ribbon and tie it in a bow around the top. Reaffirm your intention and recite the following:

> Money flows, steady to me.
> As my will, so mote it be.

6. Place your jar on your altar or in a place where you will see it regularly to keep your money goals clear in your mind.

Gratitude Ritual for Abundance

You can't ask the universe to provide you with more when you never express gratitude or appreciation for what you already have. The wise witch knows that expressing gratitude is a positive action and that positivity breeds positivity. Life provides much to be grateful for, and you mustn't let the gratitude get lost along the way.

Materials to Gather

- 1 stick basil incense for love, hope, and optimism
- Piece of paper and a pen
- Small wooden box
- 1 rhodochrosite stone for gratitude
- 1 amethyst stone for positivity
- 1 clear quartz stone for awareness

1. Cleanse, ground, and center as needed.

2. Position yourself comfortably in a quiet space, take three deep breaths, and light your incense.

3. Take your piece of paper and pen. Think about all that you have in your life. Really dig down deep and make a list of everything that comes to mind (for example, your health, home, friends, family, coven; the sun; anything you can think of that you're grateful for).

4. While making your list, allow yourself to feel whatever emotion each item brings to you (happiness, joy, peace, love, etc.). Focus on these feelings and let gratitude wash over you, filling you up from your toes to the top of your head.

5. Take your list, fold it three times, and place it inside your wooden box. Then place each crystal into the box on top of the paper one at a time.

6. Close your box securely and recite the following:

> *I am grateful and blessed for all that I have.*
> *I welcome abundance into my home.*

7. Place the box somewhere you can easily access it. Open the box and read your list or add to it whenever it feels right to do so.

CRAFTING CRYSTAL POUCHES

Crystals are a perfect magical tool to use in house magic. They have a plethora of properties to pull from and work seamlessly into any decor. The following crystal pouch recipes are for happiness, abundance, and balance—things you likely desire within your home. They are simple to make, don't require many ingredients, and can be inconspicuous in the house if necessary.

Pouch for Enhancing Happiness

Ideally, your space will be radiant and share happy and joyful energies with all who enter. If your home incites happiness, that will reflect on your own emotional wellness and overall health. Bringing in a few crystals that hold these energies is a simple and effective way to enhance the desired energies throughout your magical space.

Materials to Gather

- 1 yellow candle for joy
- 1 rose quartz stone for love
- 1 citrine stone for optimism
- 1 clear quartz stone for happiness
- Small yellow pouch for joy
- 1 drop ylang-ylang essential oil for harmony

Steps to Take

1. Cleanse, ground, and center as needed.

2. Find a space you are comfortable in and where you will not be disturbed. Sit comfortably and light your candle.

3. Clear your mind of any outside noise. Focus your thoughts on feelings of happiness and joy, those positive vibrations you would like to feel inside your home.

4. Add each stone into your pouch individually and recite the following lines for each individual stone as you place them into the pouch:

Rose quartz, bring love into this home.
Citrine, bring optimism into this home.
Clear quartz, bring happiness into this home.

5. Now take your essential oil, place one drop inside the pouch, and tie it up.

6. Hold the pouch out in front of you and recite the following:

> *Happiness will reign within these walls,*
> *Mother Goddess, hear my call.*
> *Love and joyful energies,*
> *as my will, so mote it be.*

7. You may now extinguish your flame. Place this pouch in the most frequented room of your home. You may craft more than one pouch if you think additional spaces would benefit from having one.

Pouch for Boosting Abundance

Surrounding yourself with feelings of abundance can bring to you a sense of peace of mind and calm. The energies imbued in this crystal pouch will align the energies of your home to be harmonious and welcoming to abundance in your space.

Materials to Gather

- 1 green candle for abundance, prosperity, and wealth
- 1 green aventurine stone for opportunity
- 1 moonstone for harmony
- 1 pyrite stone for good fortune
- Small green pouch for wealth
- 1 drop sandalwood essential oil for abundance and purification

Steps to Take

1. Cleanse, ground, and center as needed.

2. Find a space you are comfortable in and where you will not be disturbed. Sit comfortably and light your candle.

3. Clear your mind of any outside noise. Focus your thoughts on being open and worthy to abundance in your home. You are deserving of all that you desire.

4. Add each stone into your pouch individually and recite the following lines for each individual stone as you place them into the pouch:

> *Green aventurine, bring opportunity into this home.*
> *Moonstone, bring harmony into this home.*
> *Pyrite, bring good fortune into this home.*

5. Now take your essential oil, place one drop inside the pouch, and tie it up.

6. Hold the pouch out in front of you and recite these lines:

> *Abundance will reign within these walls,*
> *Mother Goddess, hear my call.*

Successes and prosperity, as my will, so mote it be.

7. You may now extinguish your flame. Place this pouch in the room of your home where you work on your finances and pay your bills. You may craft more than one pouch if you think additional spaces would benefit from having one.

Pouch for Harmonious Balance

It is extremely important to your overall wellness that you have a harmonious balance in the space where you spend so much of your time. A balancing ritual is wonderful to perform, but having a crystal pouch or two within your space can assist with maintaining balance in between those ritual times.

Materials to Gather

- 1 blue candle for peace and tranquility
- 1 turquoise stone for balance
- 1 lapis lazuli stone for insight
- 1 hematite stone for grounding
- Small blue pouch for harmony
- 1 drop lemongrass essential oil for balance and positivity

Steps to Take

1. Cleanse, ground, and center as needed.

2. Find a space you are comfortable in and where you will not be disturbed. Sit comfortably and light your candle.

3. Clear your mind of any outside noise. Focus your energy on finding balance within yourself. Bring this centeredness and calm into your spell work and into your home.

4. Add each stone into your pouch individually and recite the following lines for each individual stone as you place them into the pouch:

> *Turquoise, bring balance into this home.*
> *Lapis lazuli, bring insight into this home.*
> *Hematite, ground this home.*

5. Now take your essential oil, place one drop inside the pouch, and tie it up.

6. Hold the pouch out in front of you and recite these words:

> *Balance within these walls,*
> *Mother Goddess, hear my call.*
> *Insightful and grounding energies,*
> *as my will, so mote it be.*

7. You may now extinguish your flame. Place this pouch in the first room of your home. It's beneficial to make two of these so you may place one in the back room of the home as well.

Mists will last a while depending on how often you use them. They are economical, free from magic-muting toxins, and great air fresheners. For each of these three magical mists, you will require the following:

- **4-ounce dark glass spray bottle:** the dark glass is to preserve the integrity of the essential oils. Sunlight can damage the oils and can also erode certain materials over time. If you can't find a dark glass bottle, don't let that deter you; any spray bottle will do in a pinch.

- **Small stainless steel funnel:** the funnel will enable you to pour the liquids into the bottle with little to no mess.

- **½ teaspoon measuring spoon:** for measuring out the vegetable glycerin.

- **1 marked glass measuring cup:** for measuring out your liquids.

- **Witch hazel:** helps to combine the water and oils and increases the scent's staying power. Witch hazel also carries the properties of light, love, hope, and protection.

- **Distilled water:** it is pure and less likely to leave water spots on things when sprayed.

- **Vegetable glycerin:** used as a stabilizer.

Relaxation Magical Mist

When a space feels tense, it directly affects the way your physical self reacts in that space. A tense atmosphere may manifest in the body as anxiety, headaches, or fatigue and is not conducive to your witchcraft workings. This spray is wonderful for a quick refresh of a space and minimizing these symptoms.

Materials to Gather

- ½ teaspoon vegetable glycerin
- 4-ounce dark glass spray bottle
- 15 drops lemongrass essential oil for cleansing
- 9 drops neroli essential oil for relaxation
- 6 drops ylang-ylang essential oil for calm
- 2 tablespoons witch hazel
- ⅓ cup distilled water

Steps to Take

1. Cleanse, ground, and center as needed.

2. Choose your workspace. Making this mist in the kitchen is good for easy cleanup and access to tools, but you may choose wherever suits you.

3. Clear your mind of any outside noise. Let go of stresses or tensions you are holding. Your energy should match that which you are trying to manifest (in this case, relaxation).

4. Add the vegetable glycerin into the bottle first.

5. Then add in each oil individually and recite the following lines for each individual oil as you add them into the bottle:

> *Lemongrass, cleanse this space.*
> *Neroli, relax this space.*
> *Ylang-ylang, calm this space.*

6. Now add in the witch hazel and water, then place the cap on.

7. Shake the bottle and recite the following:

> *Tensions eased, stress be gone.*
> *Relax this space before too long.*
> *Calm and grounded like a tree.*
> *As my will, so mote it be.*

8. Spray three times whenever you feel the energy in a room is stressed or high-strung to enhance feelings of relaxation and peace. Always shake before using to ensure ingredients are properly mixed. Separation is natural.

Energizing Magical Mist

Occasionally you may require a little pick-me-up, and so does the energy in your home. The energies or air may begin to feel heavy, stagnant, or humid. These can be draining and leave you feeling tired, unmotivated, and in no state for performing spells or rituals. This mist is essential to energize your home.

Materials to Gather

- ½ teaspoon vegetable glycerin
- 4-ounce dark glass spray bottle
- 15 drops grapefruit essential oil for uplifting
- 9 drops lemon essential oil for joy
- 6 drops peppermint essential oil for energy
- 2 tablespoons witch hazel
- ⅓ cup distilled water

Steps to Take

1. Cleanse, ground, and center as needed.

2. Choose your workspace. Making this mist in the kitchen is good for easy cleanup and access to tools, but you may choose wherever suits you.

3. Clear your mind of any outside noise. Let go of any stresses or tensions you are holding. Try and hold feelings of optimism, joy, and vitality in your heart.

4. Add the vegetable glycerin into the bottle first.

5. Then add in each oil individually and recite the following lines for each individual oil as you add them into the bottle:

Grapefruit, uplift this space.
Lemon, bring joy to this space.
Peppermint, energize this space.

6. Now add in the witch hazel and water, then place the cap on.

7. Shake the bottle and recite the following:

Lift this space and raise it up.
Energy to fill its cup.
Joyful and flowing like the sea.
As my will, so mote it be.

8. Spray three times whenever you feel a room needs a little revitalization to help clear away any heaviness that may be dragging the energy down. Always shake before using to ensure ingredients are properly mixed. Separation is natural.

Cleansing Magical Mist

You may not always have time to perform a full cleansing ritual, or sometimes a thorough cleansing isn't entirely needed, but perhaps an argument occurred in a particular room or you had an unwanted visitor. This spray is great for quickly vanquishing negative vibes out of an area.

Materials to Gather

- ½ teaspoon vegetable glycerin
- 4-ounce dark glass spray bottle
- 10 drops lavender essential oil for peace
- 9 drops lime essential oil for cleansing
- 6 drops vanilla essential oil for love
- 2 tablespoons chamomile water for purification
- 2 tablespoons witch hazel
- 3 tablespoons distilled water

Steps to Take

1. Cleanse, ground, and center as needed.

2. Choose your workspace. Making this mist in the kitchen is good for easy cleanup and access to tools but you may choose wherever suits you.

3. Clear your mind of any outside noise. Breathe deep and allow any negativity to exhale out of your body. You should feel free of any unwanted energies.

4. Add the vegetable glycerin into the bottle first.

5. Then add in each oil individually and recite the following lines for each individual oil as you add them into the bottle:

Lavender, bring peace into this space.
Lime, cleanse this space.
Vanilla, bring love into this space.

6. Now add in the chamomile water, witch hazel, and distilled water. Place the cap on.

7. Shake the bottle and recite the following:

> *With each and every spray, negativity, please go away.*
> *Release this space and set it free.*
> *As my will, so mote it be.*

8. Spray three times whenever you feel a room has accumulated bad energy or negative vibrations. Always shake before using to ensure ingredients are properly mixed. Separation is natural.

Herb sachets can be made for a plethora of different goals, and placing them around the home is a great way to help encourage energy shifts in your space. Be sure to use dried herbs so that they will last longer than a few days. Burning a corresponding incense while crafting the sachets helps to add extra energy to the work and shift your mood into the correct mind frame.

Enhancing Positive Energies at Home

Ideally, your home environment will be a positive one, which will have a strong effect on your mood and overall well-being. Pessimistic and negative energies inside the home can lay a heavy burden on your motivations, overall outlook, and ability to perform positive magic. This sachet will help to bolster the overall feelings of positivity within the home.

Materials to Gather

- 1 stick vetiver incense to encourage positivity
- 1 tablespoon dried chamomile for harmony
- 1 tablespoon dried nettle for happiness
- 1 tablespoon dried basil for optimism and hope
- Mortar and pestle
- Small orange pouch for optimism and encouragement

Steps to Take

1. Cleanse, ground, and center as needed.

2. Find a space where you feel relaxed and will not be disturbed. This could be at your altar, your kitchen, or other space you like to perform your magical work.

3. Sit comfortably to promote a sense of calm and light your incense.

4. Clear your head and focus your mind on feelings of positivity, encouragement, and joy that you want to invite into your home.

5. Add in each herb individually to your mortar and begin blending

them together. Visualize positivity flowing through your home like a brilliant yellow thread of light affecting every area it touches.

6. Once the herbs are blended, pour them into your pouch and tie it up.

7. Hold the sachet to your heart and recite the following:

Positivity will reign within these walls,

Mother Earth, hear my call. Happy and harmonious energies, as my will, so mote it be.

8. Allow your incense to burn down fully if safe to do so. Place this sachet in the room of your home that will best be served by it. If you're not sure, the front room or most used room are good ideas.

Creating a Loving Home

Feeling love within yourself and your home is essential for achieving a healthy holistic self. Whether it be self-love or love for your partner, pets, or family members, this emotion is scientifically proven to improve overall well-being. It will also be beneficial to your magical workings. Craft this sachet with love in your heart.

Materials to Gather

- 1 stick peppermint incense for happiness
- 1 tablespoon dried rosemary for love
- 1 tablespoon dried lemon balm for purification
- 1 tablespoon dried hibiscus for passion
- Mortar and pestle
- Small pink pouch for love, friendship, and romance

Steps to Take

1. Find a space where you feel relaxed and will not be disturbed. Sit comfortably, steady your breathing, and light your incense.

2. Clear your mind and focus your mind on feelings of love: love for yourself, love for your family, love for nature, love for your home, or love for whatever ignites this feeling in you.

3. Add in each herb individually to your mortar and begin blending

them together. Visualize love flowing through your home like a glorious pink thread of light filling up every area it touches.

4. Once the herbs are blended, pour them into your pouch and tie it up.

5. Hold the pouch to your heart and recite these words:

*Love will reign within these walls,
Mother Earth, hear my call.*

*Pure and honest energies,
as my will, so mote it be.*

6. Allow your incense to burn down fully if safe to do so. Place this pouch in the kitchen, which is the heart of the home, or you can place it in whatever room you feel will most benefit from this extra loving energy. Feel free to craft more than one to be placed throughout the home as you feel appropriate.

Building a Peaceful Home

A peaceful home is a magical home. Your home is your sanctuary, and instilling feelings of peace, calm, and relaxation is incredibly important for the wellness of your environment. Promoting an atmosphere that is calm also lends itself well to being able to stay grounded and balanced in your spells and rituals.

Materials to Gather

- 1 stick lavender incense to encourage peace and relaxation
- 1 tablespoon dried lavender for peace
- 1 tablespoon dried valerian for harmony
- 1 tablespoon dried thyme for healing
- Mortar and pestle
- Small blue pouch for tranquility and calm

Steps to Take

1. Cleanse, ground, and center as needed.

2. Find a space where you feel relaxed and will not be disturbed. Sit comfortably and light your incense.

3. Clear your mind, breathe deep, slow your heart rate, relax your shoulders, and try to feel a sense of calm washing over you.

4. Add in each herb individually to your mortar and begin blending them together. Visualize peace and harmony flowing through your home like a soothing blue sphere of light reaching every inch of your space.

5. Once the herbs are blended, pour them into your pouch and tie it up.

6. Hold the pouch to your heart and recite:

Peace will reign within these walls,
Mother Earth, hear my call.
Calm and relaxed energies,
as my will, so mote it be.

7. Allow your incense to burn down fully if safe to do so. Place this pouch in the central room of your home or craft many if you wish to place around the home.

ESSENTIAL OIL MAGIC FOR THE HOME

Aromatherapy is an age-old holistic remedy and one witches have fully embraced. Aromatherapy has also gained mainstream popularity over the last few years and with good reason. The benefits are endless, such as promoting relaxation, encouraging restful sleep, and easing pain. Here are a few great ways to diffuse essential oils in your space:

- **Reusable cotton rounds:** Simply add 5–10 drops of the desired oils onto the pads and place in the appropriate areas of your home.

- **Baking soda jar:** Fill an 8- or 16-ounce Mason jar halfway with baking soda and add about 10–15 drops of the essential oil. You can either keep the lid on and open it up when you would like to use it or poke holes in the lid so that the scent will always be emitting. When the scent begins to fade, simply add more oil.

- **Eco-friendly essential oil diffuser:** It's a very effective method to get the scents of the oils wafting throughout the home in minutes. The amount of oil depends on your diffuser size. Generally accepted amounts are 3–5 drops per 100 milliliters of water it holds.

- **Reed stick diffuser:** Get a glass bottle or jar (one with a narrow top works best) and fill with ½ cup of carrier oil. Add 30 drops of your desired essential oils and stir to mix the oils together. Insert 5–8 reed sticks into the bottle. Flip the reeds after one hour to saturate the other end. To keep the scent fresh, flip the sticks one time per week.

If you have pets in the home remember to be mindful when choosing which oils to work with and how exactly you do so as some essential oils are toxic to pets. Oils such as eucalyptus, tea tree, pine, some citrus, ylang-ylang, cinnamon, and wintergreen can be harmful if applied to pets' skin, licked up, or diffused. Some safer choices include chamomile, rosemary, frankincense, and lavender. It is wise to always check with your veterinarian to be safe prior to use.

The following recipe blends encourage desirable energies throughout the home. For each one, the exact amount of each oil will depend on your chosen diffuser method.

You may make the following blends in batches to have them premixed and ready whenever you need them. This works well for blends that you know you love and will use all of the time. If you're trying new blends or just want to make one particular blend as you go, that is okay too.

Playfulness Blend

If you'd like to lighten the energy in your home and bring in some playful vibes full of freedom and cheer, then this blend will be perfect for you.

Materials to Gather

- 2 parts lemongrass essential oil for positivity
- 1 part grapefruit essential oil for freedom
- 1 part neroli essential oil for joy

Steps to Take

1. Cleanse, ground, and center as needed.

2. Choose your diffuser method.

3. Set your intentions for the blend clearly in your mind. Focus on feeling carefree, light, and happy.

4. Add each oil one at a time and recite the following:

*Lift the air and fill this space,
cheerful, light, and free.
A place for fun and joy,
true and brightened it shall
be.*

5. Spend a moment appreciating the scents. Let the oils work their magic, and surrender to those childlike feelings of carefree energy.

Focus Blend

This blend is wonderful for the work-from-home witch or those who have a home office. The properties enable the energy of the room to be motivating, focused, and clear. This will help you to make the most of your time spent there. It will also relax your nervous system and encourage you to have more self-confidence and a more positive outlook. This sense of ease and achievement will boost confidence for your magical work too.

Materials to Gather

- 2 parts sweet orange essential oil for success
- 1 part lemon essential oil for energy
- 1 part vanilla essential oil for mental clarity

Steps to Take

1. Cleanse, ground, and center as needed.

2. Choose your diffuser method.

3. Set your intentions for the blend clearly in your mind. Visualize yourself working, being productive and efficient, and getting many tasks checked off of your to-do list. Keep this picture in your mind while you blend.

4. Add each oil one at a time and recite the following:

Productivity throughout the day, every success will come my way. Motivation flow fast to me, through peace and mindful energy.

5. Spend a moment appreciating the scents. Let the oils work their magic. Tune in to your space and feel the vibrations within becoming clear, focused, and determined.

Detox Blend

This blend does wonders when something negative occurs in your space. It is beneficial when used where there was a disagreement, you received some bad news, or illness was present, and it may also be used for cleansing an area prior to performing your magical work. It is a simple way to help clear out any unsavory energies that may be lingering.

Materials to Gather

- 2 parts lemon essential oil for cleansing
- 1 part eucalyptus essential oil for banishing
- 1 part peppermint essential oil for renewal

Steps to Take

1. Cleanse, ground, and center as needed.

2. Choose your diffuser method.

3. Set your intentions for the blend clearly in your mind. Picture your space getting a sort of energy reset; envision the unwanted energies as a gray smoke being pulled out of the space and replaced by a sparkling white light. This light energy is what will remain in the space once you finish.

4. Add each oil one at a time and recite the following:

   Toxic vibes leave this space.
   Be banished to the dark.
   Cleansed, renewed, and fully free.
   A brand-new type of spark.

5. Spend a moment appreciating the scents. Let the oils work their magic. Embrace the calm, positive, and balanced energies that begin to fill your space.

CHAPTER THREE

Magic for Physical Wellness

Your physical body is your sacred vessel anchoring the spirit to this physical plane of existence. This gives your physical self a very important job to do, and it should be tended to and cared for in a manner that honors this. There are four things that everyone needs to thrive where their physical health is concerned: movement, hydration, proper nutrition, and rest. If any of these elements are lacking, your body will begin to display symptoms of distress and the potency of your magical work will also suffer. Integrating your witchcraft practice into these four areas of your life can help you take control of your physical self, allowing it to grow stronger, more connected to your mind and spirit, and more capable of producing powerful magic.

When you think of being well or "healthy," often what comes to mind first is the physical self. Do you feel energetic moving through your day? Are you free of unpleasant physical symptoms? While your physical self is not able to thrive without a healthy mind and spirit, symptoms of imbalances in the body are often first noticed as physical ones. This is your body telling you something isn't right.

This chapter will discuss how to tune in to your physical self, the connections between magic and your physical body, nutrition, and holistic rituals and remedies that will help bring your body's physical systems into a balanced state of wellness.

Really being in tune with yourself and the way your body responds to different situations is a special type of magic. Witches who are very in tune with their physical selves are able to feel how their ritual work affects them on a physical level. They are aware of certain vibrations and reactions the body has in response to their ritual and spell work. Experiencing these sensations during your witchcraft practice brings you to an ethereal level of connection with your magical workings.

Tuning in to your body and the signals it sends you, becoming connected to the energies and workings within it, is a necessary step in your magical wellness journey. The following ritual will provide you with one way to do this.

Ritual to Tune In to Your Physical Self

Taking time each day to connect with your physical self will allow you to more easily identify when something feels off. Paying attention to things such as your digestive, menstrual, and sleep patterns, along with completing this ritual, will help you to better understand your physical body. This ritual may be completed in 5 minutes or a full 30 minutes if you wish. As you become more comfortable, you will be able to move through the steps faster and with greater ease.

Materials to Gather

- 1 stick rosemary incense for clarity
- 1 blue candle for insight
- 1 amethyst stone for wisdom
- 1 clear quartz stone for awareness

Steps to Take

1. Cleanse, ground, and center as needed.

2. Choose a quiet space where you will not be disturbed. Relax and let your mind be at ease.

3. Position yourself comfortably, light your incense and say, "Sacred rosemary, bring me clarity of mind."

4. Now light your candle and say, "Healing flame and calming blue, bring insight to my spirit."

5. Pick up the amethyst stone and hold it in your right hand. Say, "Amethyst, bring me wisdom of my body within."

6. Pick up the clear quartz stone and hold it in your left hand. Say, "Clear quartz, bring me awareness of my physical self." Continue to hold both stones for the remainder of the ritual.

7. Close your eyes and bring awareness to the tips of your toes. Move and wiggle them, noticing the sensations as you do this. Then move on to your feet; move, point, and flex them, acknowledging what feels nice or not so nice. Continue this process for each part of the body: legs, abdomen, chest, arms, hands, fingers, neck, and head. For each, focus your awareness only on that one part.

8. Once you have completed this scan, bring your focus to your center. Bring your awareness to your internal systems; notice your heartbeat, how your stomach is feeling, and any sensations standing out to you. Stay in this space until you feel you have thoroughly completed this step and are feeling familiar with each part of your most inner physical self.

9. Now open your eyes, focus on your flame, and place your hands on your chest center. Recite the following:

> *I am thankful for this vessel, greater than any wealth.*
> *I will treat you well and show honor to thyself.*
> *Within and without, aware I fully see.*
> *Pure and complete, a sacred part of me.*

10. Give one final thanks to your physical self for all it does for you each day. You may now extinguish your flame and incense or allow them to burn down if able to do so safely.

Moving your body each day will ensure a proper flow and release of energies. When you don't move your body regularly, energies become stagnant and trapped, and blockages can occur. Movement helps allow these energies to move freely. It also releases negativity and creates new positive energies that will manifest as joy, motivation, and confidence. Creating this positive energy through movement will translate into better flow within your magical practice and other areas of your life.

Making a point to move every day will be a critical step on your magical wellness journey. Schedule time to do this ritual in the morning, if possible, as movement and magic are a wonderful way to start your day.

Morning Ritual to Boost Energy

Starting your day with even just a few minutes of exercise will help prepare your entire self for a more successful day. It will wake up your muscles, get your circulatory and lymphatic systems moving, elevate your mood, encourage alertness, and get your energy (including your magical energy) flowing. Aim for at least a 15-minute session each morning. That said, if there are days you can do only 5 minutes, do them! Something is better than nothing.

1. First, choose your workout ahead of time so you're prepared in the morning. This can be anything, but be sure it's something you are excited about and that will feel right for your body. Take a brisk walk, go through a yoga sequence, do an upper body workout, or dance around your living room. You can pick anything that gets you excited!

2. Next, prepare yourself and your space. While these suggestions aren't essential, they will add extra magical energy to the practice. Try utilizing crystals; bloodstone, carnelian, and tiger's eye are wonderful paired with workouts. You could have them surrounding your space, in your pocket, or worn as

comfortable jewelry. If you're able to do so safely, light a red candle to symbolize vitality and health. Lastly, dab a bit of magic-infused anointing oil on your wrists (citrus essential oil diluted with a carrier oil is great for this!) and wear a color that makes you feel strong and confident.

3. To begin, take a few deep breaths. Clear your mind of any daily commitments. This ritual is all about doing something for your health and wellness. Movement itself is a magical act; embrace it and be present in each moment.

4. As you begin to move, feel your muscles working and blood pumping with each motion. Don't rush.

Enjoy having this time to connect with your physical self.

5. Throughout the ritual, visualize yourself as strong, healthy, and thriving. You can also imagine your cells as tiny little lights zipping around your body, performing their jobs with the utmost efficiency. In this moment, you're creating positive active change.

6. Once complete, close your eyes and again take a few deep breaths. Give thanks to your body, acknowledge that vibrant energy you've awakened, and say, "Bright energy, flow strong and free. As my will, so mote it be."

Don't feel you have to complete the same activity each day. Change it up and add variety! The positive changes you experience, both physically and magically, will make it easy to keep the momentum going.

Water is a magical element and vital aspect of your life force that you are connected to every moment of the day. It flows within you and keeps you functioning. The more you move, the more hydration your body is going to require. When you move, you sweat and your body loses water. This loss must be replenished along with your basic daily hydration needs. When you aren't drinking enough water, your body will let you know it. Symptoms such as low energy, skin issues, headaches, and sugar cravings will present themselves. Feeling tired, hungry, or irritable in the afternoon? You may just be dehydrated.

Amplifying your connection to the water element with magical intention as you drink it will enable you to stay hydrated and manifest the many properties of this magical element within yourself. Your physical self and the energy you create will be more joyful, pure, flexible, and harmonious.

Connect with the Water Element

Spending a few minutes each day to connect with the water element that allows your body to function is a worthwhile venture. If we are lucky to have instant access to this life-giving force whenever we want it, it's wise to acknowledge this gift. The connected witch knows to give thanks and appreciation for the earth's resources.

Materials to Gather	Steps to Take
• Glass of drinking water	1. Cleanse, ground, and center as needed.
	2. Sit comfortably in your sacred space and set your glass of water in front of you.
	3. Close your eyes, clear your mind, and think of how amazing this element truly is. Think of the

earth's vast oceans, flowing rivers, and immense seas, and the life that lives beneath their surfaces; the water spirits that roam free; and the water that flows within yourself.

4. Open your eyes, place both of your hands above the glass, focus on the liquid within, and recite the following:

Flowing water, hydrate me.
Pure and fluid energy.
Connect me from my cells
within to vibrant sea.
As my will, so mote it be.

5. Now pick up your glass and drink the water. Feel the coolness trickle down your throat as you swallow. Feel the energy in your belly growing strong and vibrant the more you drink. Let the feeling of hydration wash over you.

6. Once you finish the glass, thank the water element for this gift.

You can complete this ritual one time per day when you are hydrating. You can also perform this while on the go as long as you're able to keep appreciation and mindfulness present. As time goes on, you will feel your connection to the water element growing within yourself, becoming stronger and easier to access. The results of this deeper connection will manifest in more vibrant physical health and success in your magical practice.

The importance of nutrition for your physical self, and for your magic, cannot be emphasized enough. The saying "you are what you eat" is truer than you may think. The foods you eat can either nourish you, making it easier for your body to thrive, or they can discourage you by adding to your body's toxicity levels.

We all have a limit to how many toxins our bodies can intake before they just can't keep up anymore and mistakes start to get made at the cellular level. A healthy body will be able to catch and fix these mistakes, but when you get run-down, things start to get missed. This is when illness and disease can form. This buildup of toxins also blocks your body's energies from flowing freely. When your body is weighed down by toxins, your magic will also feel this way. These blockages will mute the connections between your body and your magic, making it much harder to provide the appropriate energies for successful magical work.

When you choose good-quality whole foods from the earth, you will be feeding yourself essential vitamins, minerals, and earth energy with every bite you take. This will begin to clear away these excess toxins, giving your cells the best chance at thriving and your magic the best chance to blossom and grow.

Embracing seasonal whole foods will not only provide your body with everything it needs to be healthy and strong but will also strengthen your connection to the earth and the land that is local to you. When you eat foods fresh from the earth, you are taking in the energies of that food and making a sacred connection to the earth and land it was grown in. These energies can be used to benefit you in many ways, including encouraging abundance, happiness, love, success, and a more vibrant holistic self. Appreciating, giving thanks, and connecting to your food and the energies it holds is an important part of your magical wellness journey and an integral part of being a witch.

The following recipes are filled with wonderful benefits, both magical and practical, to help you on this journey. While you are cooking, you may wish to add extra magical touches to your space such as an appropriate-colored candle or crystals that align with your intentions.

The following recipes are all vegan, but if you do eat animal products, feel free to make the appropriate substitutions. The recipes will work just as well.

<<<-

Morning Magic Green Smoothie for Success
Serves 1

Getting some greens in before 9 a.m. is a definite win when it comes to your magical wellness. This smoothie contains fiber, healthy fats, vitamins C and K, iron, and calcium. It's also imbued with energies that will help set you up for a beneficial day, such as success, prosperity, love, luck, strength, and perseverance. It is especially effective when blended on a Sunday. Sunday, being ruled by the Sun, provides strong influence when it comes to success magic.

Materials to Gather

- ½ cup nondairy milk of your choice
- ½ cup filtered water
- 1 medium banana, peeled
- 2 teaspoons all-natural almond butter
- 1 tablespoon quick oats
- ½ teaspoon Ceylon cinnamon
- 1 scoop vegan vanilla protein powder (optional)
- Handful of spinach, kale, or bok choy
- 2 ice cubes

Steps to Take

1. Add all ingredients into a blender in the order listed. As you are adding each ingredient, concentrate on what the ingredients are going to do for you. They are providing you vital nutrients to nourish your body as well as motivating and energetic energies to help jump-start your day. Envision yourself going through your day being happy, productive, and the best version of yourself.

2. Hold this vision of your successful day in your mind and blend 30–60 seconds.

3. Pour blended mixture into your glass and recite the following:

Success and luck will come my way.
Prosperity and joy throughout the day.

4. Give thanks to the earth for this nourishing beverage and enjoy!

When buying protein powder, ensure that it is of high quality. The protein powder here is optional. If you don't want to include it, use ½ teaspoon pure vanilla extract and 1-2 pitted dates instead for that lovely vanilla flavor.

Blueberry Bran Muffins for Grounding

Serves 12

These healthy little muffins will delight your taste buds and magical senses. They are packed with essential nutrients such as fiber, antioxidants, potassium, and selenium. And they are rich in magical properties that will bring grounding, stability, and strength to your day.

Materials to Gather

- 1½ cups whole-wheat flour
- 1½ cups wheat bran
- ½ cup coconut sugar
- 1½ teaspoons baking soda
- 1½ teaspoons baking powder
- ½ teaspoon Ceylon cinnamon
- ½ teaspoon sea salt
- 1 flax "egg" or egg replacer (such as Bob's Red Mill)
- ¼ cup pure maple syrup
- ¾ cup unsweetened applesauce
- ¾ cup nondairy milk
- 1 tablespoon fresh lemon juice
- 1 teaspoon pure vanilla extract
- 1 cup fresh or frozen blueberries

Steps to Take

1. Prepare and cleanse your workspace. You may burn a green candle as you work to encourage balance.

2. Preheat oven to 350°F. Place compostable muffin liners into a muffin pan. While completing these steps, clear your mind and focus on your magical intentions for these muffins. Keep your intentions at the front of your mind for the entire process. Focus on the energy in your body becoming grounded and balanced.

3. In a large bowl, mix all the dry ingredients. Stir clockwise for positive encouragement to bring forth your intentions into reality. Set aside.

4. In a small bowl, mix the flax "egg" or egg replacer. Set aside to let thicken.

5. In a separate large bowl, mix all wet ingredients, adding the "egg" in last.

6. Add the wet ingredients into the dry and mix until well combined. While mixing, visualize yourself as grounded, balanced, and strong, moving through your day calmly and free from anxiety.

7. Gently fold the blueberries into the batter.

8. Fill muffin cups with batter about ⅔ of the way full. With a pointed knife, trace a pentacle, or symbol of your choosing, on the top of each muffin before placing them into the oven. Recite the following:

Nourish me and feed me well. Bring me stability and balance with this spell.

9. Bake 18–22 minutes. You will know they are finished when a toothpick inserted into the center comes out clean.

10. Remove from oven and let cool in pan 5–10 minutes.

11. Remove muffins from pan and let cool completely on a wire rack (about 60 minutes). Give thanks to the earth for this sustenance and try not to eat them all at once.

Mixing a flax "egg" is easy. Simply mix 1 tablespoon ground flax meal with 3 tablespoons water and let sit for a few minutes to thicken. These measurements will replace 1 egg in a recipe. If you need to replace 2 eggs, simply double these measurements.

Cinnamon Cacao Granola for Prosperity

Yields 3 cups

Oats are a magical food, both for your health and your witchcraft practice. Oats represent prosperity, wealth, and abundance. Eating them will enable you to utilize these energies to help maintain a prosperous mindset. They also pack a good nutritional punch with their fiber, protein, iron, and B vitamins.

Materials to Gather

- 2 cups old-fashioned rolled oats
- ½ cup raw cashew pieces
- ¼ cup raw pumpkin seeds
- ¼ cup hemp seeds
- ¼ cup unsweetened dried cranberries
- 2 tablespoons pure cacao powder
- 1½ teaspoons Ceylon cinnamon
- ½ teaspoon sea salt
- 2 tablespoons virgin coconut oil
- 3 tablespoons pure maple syrup
- 2 teaspoons pure vanilla extract

Steps to Take

1. Prepare and cleanse your workspace. Place three peridot stones on your countertop as you work to encourage prosperity and abundance.

2. Preheat oven to 300°F. Line a baking sheet with parchment paper.

3. In a large bowl, place all the dry ingredients and stir to combine.

4. Add coconut oil, maple syrup, and vanilla and mix until all of the dry ingredients are evenly coated. Using your hands for this part makes it easy to get a good even mix and really enables you to connect with each ingredient. As you mix, envision yourself as prosperous and easily attracting wealth. Allow yourself to embrace the magical energies of the ingredients and bring them forth into your days.

5. Spread the granola mixture out into an even layer on the prepared baking sheet.

6. Bake 8–10 minutes. Keep an eye on it so that it doesn't burn. When it's done, the mixture should no longer feel sticky.

7. Remove from the oven and allow to cool completely (about 45 minutes). Say your thanks for this gift and pour the granola into a Mason jar. It will remain fresh 2–3 weeks if stored in a cool, dry place. You can also keep it in the refrigerator if you'd like, but it's not necessary.

Dark Chocolate Peanut Butter Energy Balls for Love

Serves 24

These energy balls are the perfect treat when you need a little pick-me-up during your day or when you've just completed a particularly draining ritual. The ingredients of peanut butter, chocolate, maple syrup, cinnamon, and vanilla are all packed with love energy. These energy balls are also a great source of protein, healthy fats, and fiber, and they're a delicious way to connect with love energy, boost your mood, and recharge your energy.

Materials to Gather

- 1 cup all-natural peanut butter
- ¼ cup pure maple syrup
- 1 cup old-fashioned rolled oats
- 1 tablespoon cacao powder
- 2 tablespoons vegan mini chocolate chips
- ½ teaspoon Ceylon cinnamon
- 1 scoop vanilla or chocolate protein powder (optional)

Steps to Take

1. Prepare and cleanse your space. Allow yourself to release any negativity you may be holding on to. When you are making this recipe, you want to ensure you are connecting with the love energy of the ingredients. You may burn a pink candle to bring more love and tranquility into your space as you work your magic.

2. Line a storage container with wax paper.

3. Place all ingredients into a large mixing bowl and stir well to combine. Remember to stir clockwise, and allow yourself to feel love within yourself. Focus on things that invoke this emotion in you and have fun while you're moving through the steps.

4. The mix will be thick and sticky, so it will take a bit of effort to have it all come together. You may wish to mix with your hands for the last couple of minutes. This will create a deeper connection with the ingredients when you have direct hands-on contact.

5. Use a cookie scoop or tablespoon to scoop out the mixture and roll into balls. As you begin to scoop your energy balls, recite the following:

Sweet and caring energy, bring these traits unto me. Open my heart and relax my mind. Warmth and love are what I'll find.

6. Place the energy balls in the container, give thanks to Mother Earth, and store in the refrigerator. They will stay fresh up to 1 week. They also freeze well up to 3 months.

Lemon Tahini Salad Dressing for Protection

Serves 16

This dressing is sweet, tangy, and delightful. The tahini contains protein, healthy fats, antioxidants, phosphorous, and manganese. It's also packed with protective ingredients. Tahini is made from sesame, garlic, onion, black pepper, and salt, which are all powerful energetic protective aids. This is a great dressing to have when you are wanting to up your energetic protection fields.

Materials to Gather

- 4 tablespoons tahini
- Juice from half a lemon
- 2 tablespoons pure maple syrup
- 3 tablespoons water
- 1 teaspoon chopped garlic
- ½ teaspoon onion powder
- ½ teaspoon garlic powder
- ¼ teaspoon each salt and ground black pepper (adjust as needed)

Steps to Take

1. Prepare and cleanse your space. Try to bring relaxation and calm to your inner self and environment.

2. Add all ingredients into a medium bowl and whisk together until well combined. While you whisk, imagine these protective energies getting taken in and circulating throughout your body. They can be beautiful black or gold specks of light traveling from your toes up to the top of your head, creating powerful protective wards as they go. Visualize them protecting your mind, your cells, your heart, or whatever areas of yourself that need it most.

3. Once the ingredients are well mixed, pour the dressing into a glass container or Mason jar and place the lid on. Hold your hands over the container and recite the following:

> *May this earth's bounty protect and shield.*
> *With each stir, with each bit, this energy I wield.*

4. This will store well in the refrigerator 5–7 days.

Three-Bean Salad for Abundance

Serves 6

There are few foods that contain as much nutritional value and abundant energies as beans. Beans are an excellent source of fiber, protein, iron, and potassium. They also represent abundance, so they're an excellent food to add into your diet when you would like to encourage more of something in your life.

Materials to Gather

- 1 (15-ounce) can pinto beans, rinsed and drained
- 1 (15-ounce) can black beans, rinsed and drained
- 1 (15-ounce) can chickpeas, rinsed and drained
- 1 cup cooked corn
- 1 pint grape tomatoes, chopped
- ½ medium cucumber, peeled and chopped
- ½ medium red onion, peeled and chopped
- 1 medium avocado, peeled, pitted, and chopped
- Handful shredded cilantro

Steps to Take

1. Prepare and cleanse your workspace. Ease your mind and focus on invoking feelings of abundance within.

2. Add beans to a large salad bowl first. Next, add other ingredients to the bowl one at a time, feeling gratitude for each individual food.

3. Mix all ingredients together in a clockwise direction. As you mix, envision what you would like to manifest more of in life (confidence, money, love, etc.); whatever it may be, imagine it entering your life in new and magical ways.

4. Once the ingredients are mixed, close your eyes, place your hands above the bowl, and recite the following:

> *Sacred earth foods, nourish me well.*
> *Abundance will come, with this spell.*

5. Top with the Lemon Tahini Salad Dressing for Protection (see recipe in this chapter). This will make it a meal with abundance and protective properties in one. You may also use another of your favorite dressings if you wish. Give thanks to the earth and enjoy.

Mushroom and Greens Miso Stir-Fry for Psychic Abilities

Serves 4

As a witch, you will have times when you would like to open your mind and expand your psychic awareness, perhaps when you are working on your divination practice or developing your astral projection skills. Mushrooms, dandelion greens, edamame, and celery hold properties connected to these abilities, and ingesting them can be helpful on your path. They also have a plethora of nutrients such as vitamin A, iron, magnesium, and B vitamins. Prepare this meal on a Wednesday, ruled by Mercury, and an optimal day for divination work.

Materials to Gather

- 3 medium cloves garlic, peeled and chopped
- 1 medium red onion, peeled and chopped
- ½ cup vegetable broth
- 1 pint shiitake mushrooms, or mushrooms of your choice
- 3 medium stalks celery, chopped
- 1 cup shelled edamame (fresh or frozen)
- ½ cup frozen corn
- 1 medium bunch dandelion greens
- 2 tablespoons miso paste
- 2 tablespoons coconut aminos
- ½ teaspoon onion powder
- Pinch sea salt and ground black pepper (adjust as needed)

Steps to Take

1. Cleanse and prepare your space. Clear your mind and simply focus on the joy of creating this magical, nutritious meal.

2. In a large skillet over medium heat, add garlic, onion, and broth. Sauté 2–3 minutes.

3. Add mushrooms to pan and sauté another 2–3 minutes.

4. Stir in celery and cook until it begins to become translucent, about 3 minutes.

5. Add in edamame and corn. Cover, reduce heat to low, and let cook 3–5 minutes.

6. Add in dandelion greens. Cover and leave on low heat.

7. In a small dish, mix together miso paste, coconut aminos, and onion powder. As you mix, imagine you are creating space with this meal, opening up your mind to a universe beyond your grasp. Allow your senses to tune in to that which we cannot see.

8. Add this paste to the vegetables in the pan, sprinkle with salt and pepper, and stir well. Continue stirring for about 2 minutes while imagining your psychic abilities being elevated to new levels. Imagine yourself honing in on these skills in whatever form you would like them to manifest; whether it's tarot readings, precognition, or mediumship, envision yourself excelling at the task.

9. Once everything is mixed, you may serve immediately. It is lovely with brown rice or rice noodles. Again, be sure to give your thanks for this nourishing gift.

"Cheesy" Lentil Pasta Bake for Peace and Purity

Serves 6

Pasta is truly a feel-good food, and this pasta happens to be brimming with healthy nutrients and magical properties. From protein and iron to B vitamins and calcium, this dish has it all. Magically, it's a harmonious meal promoting peace, comfort, and purity.

Materials to Gather

- 1 (8-ounce) box red lentil pasta
- 1 cup tomato sauce
- 3 medium cloves garlic, peeled and chopped
- 1 medium onion, peeled and chopped
- ¾ cup vegetable broth, divided
- 2 cups mushrooms, chopped
- 2 cups whole green beans
- ¼ teaspoon sea salt
- ¼ teaspoon ground black pepper, plus an extra sprinkle, divided
- ¾ cup full-fat coconut cream
- 3 tablespoons nutritional yeast
- 2 tablespoons tapioca flour or cornstarch
- ½ teaspoon miso paste
- 1 teaspoon onion powder
- 1 teaspoon garlic powder
- Pinch cayenne pepper
- Small bunch fresh basil

Steps to Take

1. Prepare and cleanse your space. Allow yourself to feel a sense of calm and harmony within. Hold this feeling throughout your cooking process.

2. Preheat oven to 350°F.

3. Fill a large stockpot with 4 cups water and bring to a boil over high heat. Once it begins to boil, add pasta and cook 8–10 minutes. Drain pasta and mix in tomato sauce. Set aside when done.

4. In a medium skillet over medium heat, add garlic, onion, and ½ cup vegetable broth. Sauté 2–3 minutes.

5. Add mushrooms to pan and continue cooking for 2–3 minutes.

6. Stir in green beans, then add in salt and half of your black pepper. Cover, reduce heat to low, and cook 5 minutes.

7. While the vegetables are cooking, make the "cheese" sauce. In a medium saucepan, place coconut cream, ¼ cup vegetable broth, nutritional yeast, tapioca flour, miso paste, ¼ teaspoon black pepper, onion powder, garlic powder, and cayenne and whisk ingredients together until combined. Place the pan on the stove and turn the heat to high. Bring to a boil, then turn down heat and simmer on low. Simmer 2–3 minutes while stirring gently, allowing sauce to thicken.

8. Add vegetables into the pasta and combine.

9. Pour the pasta mixture into an ungreased 8" × 8" casserole dish.

10. Top pasta with the "cheese" sauce, a sprinkle of black pepper, basil, and vegan cheese (if using).

11. Trace the word "peace" in the air above your dish and say, "May this dish bring to me peace and comfort." Bake covered 20–25 minutes. Uncover the last 5 minutes.

12. Remove, let cool 5 minutes, give thanks to the earth, and enjoy.

THE MAGIC OF SLEEP

Proper sleep is important for a healthy holistic self. While you sleep, your body is able to rest, heal, and rejuvenate itself. It's when you are allowed to turn your mind off and get lost in magical dreams of divine forests and mystical realms.

When you don't allow your body proper time for sleep, all of your body's systems are affected. Symptoms such as fatigue, hormone imbalance, increased cravings, and weight gain may present themselves. When you are feeling drained due to lack of sleep, your witchcraft practice will also suffer as you simply won't have the proper energy to put into your spells. And if you are not preparing yourself for rest or you have an undesirable sleep environment, your body may not be getting the most out of the time you do spend sleeping. Following are some tips for better sleep habits:

- Have a sleep schedule. Go to bed and wake up at the same time each day.

- Follow the natural rhythms of the earth by going to bed early and waking with the sun.

- Diffuse essential oils that encourage sleep and calm such as lavender, chamomile, or valerian.

- Remove electronic devices from your sleeping space.

- Create a relaxing, sleep-inducing atmosphere in your bedroom. Keep it clean and uncluttered.

- Keep crystals that promote good rest, such as moonstone, celestite, or howlite.

- Keep your room as dark as possible when you're going to sleep; even the slightest bit of light can affect your sleep cycles.

- Try to spend at least 30 minutes prior to bedtime winding down with a relaxing activity that does not include the television, computer, or your phone.

- Create a bedtime routine for yourself. Have a cup of tea, read a book, pull a tarot card, perform a sleep meditation, or indulge in a relaxing ritual bath.

- Come to view your bedroom as a space for healing and relaxation.

If you are someone to whom sleep doesn't come easy, the following practices can be added to your sleep routine for some extra encouragement.

Meditation for Peaceful Rest

Performing a meditation right before dozing off can release tension in your body, ease your mind, create a deeper connection to your physical self, and affect how you dream. Meditation also activates your parasympathetic nervous system, enabling your body to become calm and allowing you to awaken properly rested.

Materials to Gather

- Yourself and your bed

Steps to Take

1. Once you are fully ready for bed, lie down comfortably and close your eyes.

2. Take a moment to relax your body and sink into your mattress. Let your mind feel at ease and let go of the day's activities, your to-do lists, or anything that may be causing you stress.

3. Take three deep breaths. Take four counts to inhale and four to exhale.

4. Focus your mind on the gift of sleep, rest, and rejuvenation for your body. It has worked hard for you during the day and deserves this break.

5. In your mind, state the following three times.

> *I will allow my body to rest.*
> *I will enjoy a good night's sleep.*
> *I will awake energetic and happy.*

6. Continue to focus on how good it feels to just let yourself be calm and quiet. Continue focusing on your deep breathing until you drift off to sleep.

Lavender Dream Pouch

Lavender is well known to induce and promote sleep. Its properties encourage peace, calm, and positive dreams. Studies have also shown lavender not only helps you fall asleep but improves the quality of sleep as well. It can have you feeling rested, energetic, and at your most magical in the morning.

Materials to Gather

- 1 stick lavender incense to promote peace
- 2 tablespoons dried lavender buds for sleep and positive dreaming
- 1 tablespoon dried valerian for sleep and harmony
- Mortar and pestle
- Small blue pouch for serenity and calm
- 1 howlite stone for relaxation
- 3 drops lavender essential oil for added aromatherapy benefits

Steps to Take

1. Cleanse, ground, and center as needed.

2. Gather ingredients and set up your workspace. Choose a quiet space you will not be disturbed. Sit comfortably to promote relaxation and light your incense.

3. Clear your head and focus your mind on getting a restful sleep; having positive, peaceful dreams; and awakening refreshed and rejuvenated.

4. Add in each herb individually to your mortar and begin blending them together. Visualize yourself sleeping soundly, relaxed, and uninterrupted for eight hours.

5. Once the herbs are blended, pour them into your pouch and add the howlite. Add in essential oil and tie it up.

6. Close your eyes, hold the pouch to your heart, and say:

> *Allow for slumber, allow for sleep.*
> *Drifting, dreaming, slow and deep.*
> *Sacred lavender, bring rest to me.*
> *As my will, so mote it be.*

7. Open your eyes, place this pouch under your favorite pillow, and enjoy the benefits of a good night's sleep. Allow your incense to burn down fully if safe to do so.

Sleep Well Magical Pillow Spray

A spray for your pillow can have the same aromatherapy effects as using a pouch or diffusing an oil blend. A spray will also emit some of the same energies into your room and surrounding sleep space. You may wish to use this spray along with our lavender dream pouch for added benefits.

Materials to Gather

- ½ teaspoon vegetable glycerin
- 4-ounce dark glass spray bottle
- 15 drops lavender essential oil for sleep
- 9 drops chamomile essential oil for calm
- 6 drops clary sage essential oil for grounding
- 2 tablespoons witch hazel
- ⅓ cup distilled water

Steps to Take

1. Cleanse, ground, and center as needed.

2. Gather ingredients and prepare your workspace. As in our other spray recipes, the kitchen works well for easy prep and cleanup.

3. Clear your mind of any outside distractions. Focus on feeling relaxed and calm, the way you would like to feel as you are drifting off to sleep.

4. Use a stainless steel funnel to add the vegetable glycerin to the bottle.

5. Then add in each oil individually and recite the following lines as you add in each individual oil to the bottle:

Lavender, bring me sleep.
Chamomile, bring me calm.
Clary sage, ground me strong.

6. Add in the witch hazel, fill the bottle with the distilled water, and place the cap on.

7. Shake the bottle and recite the following:

Send me off to dreamland.
Sleep in the palm of my hand.
Calm and grounded I shall be.
To awaken with vibrant energy.

8. Shake prior to each use and spray your pillow with three light spritzes before bed to enhance feelings of peace and promote sound sleep. Remember to be mindful of who has access to your pillow as not all essential oils are safe for pets and children.

Using herbal remedies for healing connects you with the powerful and intelligent energies contained within each plant. As a witch, you are aware of the wisdom in the earth and within the energies each plant holds. These energies can assist in enabling your body to activate its self-healing abilities. Being able to utilize and harness these energies is a gift to be thankful for.

The following recipes will help aid the body on a path toward better wellness through the power of plants. If you wish, light a blue candle for its healing energies while crafting and prepare these close to a new or full moon. New and full moons are optimal times to perform spells for health and healing; a Sunday or Monday will also work well. Both of these days lend themselves well to healing work due to their planetary associations of the Sun and Moon. For each of these remedies, please use care and check for possible interactions if you are on medication or have any illnesses.

Magical Tinctures

A tincture is an extraction of a plant's properties via alcohol. Tinctures can also be done with apple cider vinegar or vegetable glycerin, but those are less potent and the results are technically extracts, not tinctures (though they're great options for those who abstain from alcohol or young children). The following three tincture recipes, which use vodka because it does the best job of extraction, will follow the same basic steps and process. Tinctures must sit for 4–6 weeks before they are ready for use. With that in mind they are best prepared in advance so that you have them on hand when an issue arises. Craft as much as is appropriate for your needs.

Thyme Tincture for Candida

Candida is present in everyone in small amounts. Issues arise when an overgrowth occurs, which releases toxins into the body, disrupting body systems and the natural flow of energy. It's surprisingly common and can cause an array of symptoms such as fatigue, digestive upset, and irritability. An overgrowth can eventually cause more severe problems and may need medical attention, but if addressed early can be managed through diet and magical herbal aids.

Materials to Gather

- Fresh or dried thyme
- Mortar and pestle
- Mason jar
- Vodka
- Dark glass bottle

Steps to Take

1. Cleanse your space and gather all necessary ingredients. These types of herbal potions are best made in your kitchen for easy cleanup. Clear your mind and focus on the task at hand.

2. Place the thyme into your mortar and begin to crush the herb just enough to begin to release the oils; this allows for a better extraction process and stronger tincture than if the herb is left whole. This step is important particularly for fresh herbs, for dried herbs it's more symbolic. As you crush the herb, say, "Sacred thyme, lend me your healing power to cleanse candida from my body."

3. Open your Mason jar and fill no more than two-thirds of the way with the thyme.

4. Pour the vodka over the herbs to cover 2" above where they end. You want them completely covered. While pouring, imagine the candida swirling through your body and gathering into a little ball of energy, then traveling out the top of your head and dissipating into the air.

5. Secure the lid on your jar. If the lid is metal, you will want to cover the mouth of the jar with parchment paper first to prevent rusting. Give the contents a shake to mix and say, "Herb of the earth, heal me well. Candida, I release you with this spell."

6. Store your tincture in a cool, dark, and dry space for 4–6 weeks, shaking daily. Each day you go to shake your tincture, recite the same line: "Herb of the earth, heal me well. Candida, I release you with this spell." If you notice some of your alcohol has evaporated and the herbs are exposed, be sure to add a little more to prevent bacterial growth.

7. After the 4–6 weeks, once your tincture is ready you must strain the liquid. Drape a cheesecloth over a stainless steel funnel and place into your bottle. Slowly strain liquid into the funnel. Give the cheesecloth a squeeze to release every drop of the tincture. Place the cap on your bottle and thank the herbs for their service.

Take 1 teaspoon two to three times daily either on its own or diluted in water. Tinctures have a long shelf life due to the alcohol content and may last years when stored in a cool, dark, and dry space away from heat and light.

Ginger Tincture for Nausea

Ginger is widely accepted for alleviating nausea and upset stomach. There are many instances where one may experience nausea from motion sickness or stress to absorbing too much negative energy from others. Having this tincture on hand for instances such as these is practical, convenient, and will keep you from having to reach for anti-nausea medications.

Materials to Gather

- Fresh or dried ginger
- Mortar and pestle
- Mason jar
- Vodka
- Dark glass bottle

Steps to Take

1. Cleanse your space and gather all necessary ingredients. Clear your mind and focus on the task at hand.

2. Place the ginger into your mortar and begin to crush the herb, again just enough to begin to release the oils. As you crush the herb, say, "Sacred ginger, lend me your healing power to ease my nausea."

3. Open your Mason jar and add in the ginger, filling no more than two-thirds of the way.

4. Pour the vodka over the herbs to cover 2" above where they end. You want them completely covered. While pouring, imagine the ginger efficiently working its way through your system into your stomach and surrounding the nausea with a healing blue light until it shrinks down into nothing and disappears.

5. Secure the lid on your jar. If the lid is metal, you will want to cover the mouth of the jar with parchment paper first to prevent rusting. Give the contents a shake to mix and say, "Herb of the earth, heal me well. Nausea, I release you with this spell."

6. Store your tincture in a cool, dark, and dry space for 4–6 weeks, shaking daily. Each day you go to shake your tincture, say the same line: "Herb of the earth, heal me well. Nausea, I release you with this spell." If you notice some of your alcohol has evaporated and the herbs are exposed, be sure to add a little more to prevent bacterial growth.

7. After 4–6 weeks, once your tincture is ready, you must strain the liquid. Drape a cheesecloth over a stainless steel funnel and place into your bottle. Slowly strain liquid into the funnel. Give the cheesecloth a squeeze to release every drop of the tincture. Place the cap on your bottle and thank the herbs for their service.

Take 1 teaspoon when required (no more than three times daily) on its own or diluted in water. Tinctures have a long shelf life due to the alcohol content and may last years when stored in a cool, dark, and dry space away from heat and light.

Red Raspberry Leaf Tincture for Hormone Balance

Red raspberry leaf has been used for centuries to aid hormonal health. Hormones circulate throughout the body just like energy and work synergistically together to create a cohesive, well-functioning environment. An imbalance can result in many unpleasant symptoms such as irritability, poor sleep, sluggish metabolism, and spiritual energies that are out of sync, creating strife for your body systems, emotions, and magical practice.

Materials to Gather

- Fresh or dried raspberry leaf
- Mortar and pestle
- Mason jar
- Vodka
- Dark glass bottle

Steps to Take

1. Cleanse your space and gather your materials. Clear your mind and focus on the task at hand.

2. Place the red raspberry leaf into your mortar and begin to crush the herb. As you crush the herb, say, "Sacred red raspberry leaf, lend me your healing power to bring my hormones into balance."

3. Open your Mason jar and fill no more than two-thirds of the way with the red raspberry leaf.

4. Pour the vodka over the herbs to cover 2" above where they end. You want them covered completely. While pouring, imagine your hormones circulating throughout your body as glittering green lights. Imagine them traveling from your toes all the way to the top of your head in a harmonious and balanced journey. Imagine these lights creating a symmetry within yourself.

5. Secure the lid on your jar. If the lid is metal, you will want to cover the mouth of the jar with parchment paper first to prevent rusting. Give the contents a shake to mix and say, "Herb of the earth, heal me well. Balance my hormones with this spell." If you notice some of your alcohol has evaporated and the herbs are exposed be sure to add a little more to prevent bacterial growth.

6. Store your tincture in a cool, dark, and dry space for 4–6 weeks, shaking daily. Each day you go to shake your tincture, recite the same line: "Herbs of the earth, heal me well. Balance my hormones with this spell."

7. After 4–6 weeks, once your tincture is ready, you must strain the liquid. Drape a cheesecloth over a stainless steel funnel and place into your bottle. Slowly strain liquid into the funnel. Give the cheesecloth a squeeze to release every drop of the tincture. Place the cap on your bottle and thank the herbs for their service.

Take 1 teaspoon two to three times daily either on its own or diluted in water. Tinctures have a long shelf life due to the alcohol content and may last years when stored in a cool, dark, and dry space away from heat and light.

Arnica Salve for Muscle and Joint Pain

Muscle aches and strains can range from unpleasant to debilitating. This salve, with the amazing healing powers of arnica and Saint-John's-wort, is sure to ease what is ailing you. When you're having a flare-up of pain, massage this salve gently into the area. While you massage the area, visualize the healing powers of the plant ingredients working to bring the pain and inflammation to the surface of the skin and releasing it. Do keep in mind that Saint-John's-wort can make the skin oversensitive to light in some individuals. Be sure to take care and protect your skin if you will be going outside after use.

Materials to Gather

- 4 teaspoons arnica-infused oil
- 2 teaspoons avocado oil
- 2 teaspoons Saint-John's-wort–infused oil
- 1 tablespoon shea butter
- 1 teaspoon candelilla wax
- ½ teaspoon vitamin E oil
- 6 drops lavender essential oil
- 6 drops rosemary essential oil
- 2-ounce dark glass jar

Steps to Take

1. Cleanse your workspace and gather your ingredients.

2. Add about 3" worth of water in the bottom pot of a double boiler and place over low heat.

3. Add arnica-infused oil, avocado oil, Saint-John's-wort–infused oil, and shea butter to the pot. Stir the contents gently in a clockwise direction to encourage positive results until the shea butter is fully melted, about 2 minutes.

4. Add in the candelilla wax. Stir the contents gently until wax is melted, about another minute.

5. Add in vitamin E oil and stir to combine.

6. Turn off heat and add in each essential oil. Stir clockwise to combine and say:

> *Ease my aches, release my strain.*
> *Herb of arnica, dissolve my pain.*

7. Immediately pour the mixture into your jar and let cool. Ensure salve is completely cooled before placing and securing the lid.

You may apply the salve as needed. It should last up to 12 months when stored in a cool, dry place away from direct sunlight. As time passes the natural scents from the oils will begin to fade, which is normal, but if it's gone off, a rancid smell will develop.

Alternatives to using a double boiler if you don't have one is either placing a heatproof measuring cup directly into a pot of hot water or placing the right size heatproof bowl on top of your pot with hot water and then combining your ingredients in there instead. Works just as well!

Lemon Oregano Herbal Cough Syrup

Oregano is a powerful antiviral, and lemon is cleansing and very high in vitamin C, which is needed for a strong immune system. The pair works extremely well to combat common coughs and colds. When you're sick with a cold, not much is going to get done in your magical or mundane life. Keep this cough syrup on hand, especially throughout the colder months, so you may begin treating the illness straightaway.

Materials to Gather

- 3 teaspoons dried oregano
- Rind of 1 medium lemon
- 1½ cups filtered water
- 1 cup pure maple syrup (cane sugar or honey may also be used)
- Juice of 1 medium lemon
- 16-ounce Mason jar

Steps to Take

1. Cleanse your workspace and gather your ingredients.

2. Create a decoction of the oregano and lemon rind by adding these plus the water into a small saucepan pan and bringing to a boil over high heat. Turn heat down to low and let simmer for 20–30 minutes.

3. While the decoction is simmering, take this time to focus your energy on healing the body. Visualize a strong immune system efficiently combating any illness that may present itself. Envision a healing aura surrounding you, providing strength and determination to be well.

4. When the liquid is ready, strain it into a separate small saucepan. Add the maple syrup and lemon juice and bring to a boil over high heat. Turn heat down to low and allow the mixture to thicken, stirring in a clockwise direction continuously, about 5–10 minutes. If you prefer a thicker syrup, simply lessen the amount of water used.

5. Remove from heat and allow to cool completely, approximately 2 hours. Pour cooled liquid into your Mason jar and secure the lid.

This will keep up to 8 weeks stored in the refrigerator. Use personal discretion for dosage, but 1 teaspoon three times daily is a good place to start.

Lavender Eucalyptus Oil Blend for Headache Relief

Many things can contribute to headaches such as dehydration, hunger, stress, or, for empaths, being surrounded by the negative or overwhelming emotions of others. Lavender and peppermint both have uplifting properties that encourage happiness, further helping to ease your strain. This oil blend is fantastic to have on hand, and you may even wish to carry a small vile with you when you're away from home.

Materials to Gather

- 10 drops lavender essential oil
- 8 drops eucalyptus essential oil
- 4 drops peppermint essential oil
- 1-ounce dark glass dropper bottle
- ½ teaspoon vegetable glycerin
- 5 teaspoons neutral carrier oil (jojoba, sweet almond, grapeseed, coconut, or avocado)

Steps to Take

1. Cleanse your workspace and gather your ingredients.

2. Place each of the essential oils into the bottle one at a time. Say:

   Lavender, relax my mind.
   Eucalyptus, clear my head.
   Peppermint, relieve my pain.

3. Insert a funnel into your bottle and pour in the vegetable glycerin and carrier oil.

4. Securely close the top and shake the bottle for 30 seconds. Say, "Herbs of the earth, ease my mind; allow this headache to be left behind."

5. To use, you can rub a drop into each of your temples, or simply open the bottle and inhale the scents of the oils for a bit of aromatherapy. As you use the oil blend, you may wish to recite the line from step 4 and come back to your visualization. Shake before each use as separation of oils is natural. Oil blends such as this may be safely stored in a cool, dark, and dry place at least 6–12 months. Over time the scents from the oils will fade, but if you notice a rancid smell develop you will know it has gone off.

Allergies Be Gone Oil Blend

Allergies are brought on by the immune system overreacting to a normally safe substance. The immune system is related to your first energy center, located at the base of your spine, so allergies may also be a manifestation of blockages in this area. While you work to create balanced energies within, you can keep this blend on hand to help release your sinuses and ease discomfort.

Materials to Gather

- 4 drops lavender essential oil
- 4 drops lemon essential oil
- 4 drops peppermint essential oil
- 2 drops tea tree essential oil
- 1-ounce dark glass bottle
- ½ teaspoon vegetable glycerin
- 5 teaspoons neutral carrier oil (jojoba, sweet almond, grapeseed, coconut, or avocado)

Steps to Take

1. Cleanse your space and gather your ingredients.

2. Place each of the essential oils into the bottle one at a time. As you do this, imagine your allergies evaporating or being pulled out of your body. These do not serve you, and it's time to let them go. Visualize yourself breathing well and free from your unpleasant and distracting symptoms.

3. Insert a funnel into your glass bottle and pour in the vegetable glycerin and carrier oil.

4. Securely close the top and shake the bottle for 30 seconds. Say, "Herbs of the earth, release my symptoms and bring me clarity."

5. Apply this blend as needed over sinuses, above eyebrows, under nose, on the forehead, or back of the neck. As you use the oil blend, you may wish to recite the line from step 4 and come back to your visualization. Shake before each use as separation of oils is natural. Oil blends such as this may be safely stored in a cool, dark, and dry place for at least 6–12 months. Over time the scents from the oils will fade, but if you notice a rancid smell develop you will know it has gone off.

Herbal Compress for Cuts, Scrapes, and Bruises

The healing powers of chamomile, calendula, and yarrow work together in this herbal compress for use on minor cuts, scrapes, and bruises. These three plants have long been used for healing practices. They are powerful and gentle plants with relaxing and calming energies capable of creating much healing magic within the body.

Materials to Gather

- 1 stick eucalyptus incense for healing and cleansing
- 1½ cups water
- 1 tablespoon dried chamomile
- 1 tablespoon dried yarrow
- 1 tablespoon dried calendula
- Tea strainer
- Clean cloth

Steps to Take

1. Cleanse your space, gather your ingredients, and light your incense.

2. Fill a small saucepan with the water and bring to a boil over medium heat.

3. Add the herbs and steep them on low heat for 10–20 minutes.

4. While the herbs are steeping, sit with your incense for a few minutes and visualize your wounds healing quickly, revealing smooth and soft skin. Focus on the energies in these herbs helping to bring this healing into reality.

5. Once the appropriate time has passed, remove from heat and strain the liquid through a tea strainer into a glass or bowl. You may discard the herbs in the compost (if applicable).

6. Soak the clean cloth in the infused liquid and squeeze off the excess. Apply the warm cloth directly to the affected area and state the following: "Herbs of the earth, heal my wounds and ease my pain." Leave the cloth on for 10–20 minutes. You may repeat this several times per day. Simply reheat the remaining liquid and be sure to use a clean cloth each time. The remaining liquid can be kept for 2–3 days in the refrigerator if you have some left over.

Immunity-Boosting Wellness Shot

Wellness shots will give you energy, support your immune system, and give you a little jolt of nutrients and positivity. Use these shots during cold and flu season or when you're feeling run-down to help revitalize you. The ingredients, such as the lemon and orange, also contain joyful and uplifting energies for you to utilize as you move through your day. This shot is best if consumed right away.

Materials to Gather

- Juice from 1 medium lemon
- ¼ medium orange, peeled
- 1" piece ginger (no need to peel)
- 2 tablespoons coconut water
- Pinch cayenne pepper

Steps to Take

1. Cleanse your space and gather your ingredients.

2. Place all ingredients into a blender and blend until smooth.

3. Strain the mixture through a cheesecloth to clear away any remaining bits and pieces.

4. Pour the mixture into a glass and say, "Golden liquid, bring strength to my immune system and positive energy to my mind." Give thanks to the earth and enjoy!

Gut-Repairing Turmeric Latte

Turmeric is energetically protective and high in antioxidants helping the body combat free radicals, protect cells from damage, and fight off illness. Turmeric is also helpful when you're suffering regular digestive upset, possibly caused by leaky gut syndrome. Leaky gut occurs when small gaps begin to open in your intestinal walls, which allow toxins and bacteria to enter your bloodstream, resulting in many symptoms. This delicious latte can help repair your gut while providing you with energetic protection for your digestive tract.

Materials to Gather

- 1 tablespoon coconut oil
- 1 teaspoon turmeric powder
- ¼ teaspoon ground black pepper
- 1¼ cups nondairy milk (oat, soy, cashew, or almond are all good choices)
- ½ teaspoon Ceylon cinnamon
- 1 teaspoon pure vanilla extract
- 1 tablespoon pure maple syrup

Steps to Take

1. Cleanse your workspace, gather your ingredients, and clear your mind. Focus your energies on this magical beverage you are brewing and the positive effects it will have on your well-being.

2. In a small bowl, add coconut oil, turmeric powder, and pepper and mix into a paste. As you mix, envision a protective energetic lining flowing through your intestinal walls, keeping them from further harm.

3. Pour the nondairy milk into a small saucepan and turn the heat to medium.

4. Once the nondairy milk begins to warm, add in the turmeric paste, cinnamon, vanilla, and

maple syrup. Stir clockwise to encourage your desired results. As you stir, visualize your digestive tract healing and imagine any gaps within your intestinal wall closing up and repairing themselves. As these spaces repair themselves, imagine little rays of light appearing in their place, instead signaling that you are healed and well. Keep this visualization in your mind throughout the preparation and while you're drinking the beverage.

5. Once ingredients are well combined after about 3 minutes, turn off the heat and pour the latte into a mug. Say, "Magical turmeric, heal me well. Bring comfort and protection with this spell."

6. If possible, have this as a nighttime beverage. Sit somewhere comfortably to sip it and relax. Perhaps you would like to light a blue candle or lavender incense for healing as you drink. Focus on healing yourself and keeping that previous visualization in your mind.

This is also great as a morning beverage if you prefer to have it then. Have one per day to help repair your gut, improve overall digestion, and add that layer of energetic protection within.

Always be sure to include the black pepper in your Turmeric Latte recipe. Black pepper ensures better absorption of the turmeric, providing much greater benefit than if you take the turmeric alone as it is not absorbed well by the body.

Herbal magic isn't just for the inside of your body. When you feel confident on the outside, it allows for more positive energies to flow within yourself, leading to better overall physical wellness and a stronger magical practice. Crafting remedies that aid your appearance is also an opportune moment to perform some glamour magic.

Glamour magic is a shift or projection of energy relating to your appearance or aura, enhancing how others perceive you, as well as how you see yourself. Your beauty or grooming routine is a perfect time to indulge in this type of magic and give yourself a nice boost of confidence.

Skin, hair, and nails are not just about looking and feeling beautiful. They can show signs of imbalances in body systems as well. For example, eczema can be a sign of food intolerance, dry hair can signify vitamin deficiency, and brittle nails can be a sign of low iron. You ultimately want to try and keep your outside elements strong and healthy with proper nutrition, but sometimes they need a little help along the way, and the following remedies are here for you.

Witch's Water for Acne

This magical toner will cleanse, tighten, and refresh your skin. Using a toner each day will remove excess dirt from pores, help the skin retain moisture, and combat acne. These ingredients work together to create an amazing synergistic effect for your skin. The energies they contain are calming and uplifting.

Materials to Gather

- ½ teaspoon vegetable glycerin
- 4-ounce dark glass bottle
- 6 drops sweet orange essential oil
- 2 tablespoons alcohol-free witch hazel
- ¼ cup chamomile water
- 5 teaspoons lavender water

Steps to Take

1. Cleanse your workspace and gather your materials.

2. Ease your mind from any outside noise. Your energy should be focused only on what you are trying to achieve: clear and healthy skin. Visualize yourself as having perfectly clear, smooth, and nourished skin that is free from dryness, acne, or signs of fatigue. Hold this vision in your mind as you go through the mixing process. Keep your intentions very clear on the task at hand.

3. Use a funnel to add the vegetable glycerin to the bottle.

4. Add in sweet orange essential oil.

5. Add the witch hazel and chamomile and lavender waters, then place the cap on the bottle.

6. Shake the bottle and recite the following:

> Skin be cleansed, skin be clear.
> Smooth and healthy each day of the year.
> Nourished, hydrated, and acne-free.
> As my will, so mote it be.

7. Your toner is ready to use. Shake prior to each use. Apply each morning and evening with a soft cloth as part of your skin care routine for optimal results. Recite the following affirmation each time you use your new toner: "I have beautifully nourished, healthy, and clear skin."

Coconut Oat Bath for Eczema

Skin issues are often an allergic response associated to a food sensitivity. Your skin is your largest detox organ, and when toxins overburden the body, excess toxins get released through your skin, causing issues such as eczema, acne, and psoriasis. Skin issues are also one more thing that can arise due to toxic energy blockages within the body. This oat bath will help ease the uncomfortable symptoms that may present themselves.

Materials to Gather

- 2 cups old-fashioned rolled oats
- ¾ cup coconut milk powder
- ¼ cup dried calendula flowers
- 6 drops eucalyptus essential oil
- 12 drops vanilla essential oil

Steps to Take

1. Cleanse your workspace and gather your materials. Clear your mind and focus on your goal: relief from eczema and hydrated, happy skin.

2. In a medium bowl, combine all the dry ingredients. Add in each essential oil and mix well. Recite the following:

> *Skin be clear, smooth, and free from pain.*
> *Toxicity released and only healthy skin shall remain.*

3. Add ½–1 cup into a mesh bag or nylon stocking to prevent a messy tub. Drop into your bath. Soak yourself for at least 15 minutes and visualize the properties from your ingredients spreading out and enveloping any areas of eczema with a glittering, healing light. Envision your eczema fading away to reveal soft and smooth skin.

Soothing Hand Salve for Dry Skin

Many things cause dry skin, including dehydration. If your skin is excessively dry, remember to hydrate extra. In the meantime, you may utilize this soothing salve containing the incredible plant powers of calendula and aloe, both well known for their moisturizing properties. Energetically, they contain healing and protective energies that will encourage further healing of the skin.

Materials to Gather

- 4 teaspoons pumpkin seed carrier oil
- 1 tablespoon calendula-infused oil
- 1 tablespoon aloe butter
- 1 teaspoon candelilla wax
- ½ teaspoon vitamin E oil
- 4 drops lavender essential oil
- 2 drops patchouli essential oil
- 2 drops neroli essential oil
- 2-ounce dark glass jar

Steps to Take

1. Cleanse your workspace and gather your ingredients. Clear your mind and relax into the task at hand.

2. Add water to the bottom of a double boiler and turn heat to low.

3. Add pumpkin seed and calendula-infused oils to the pot, then add the aloe butter. Stir the contents gently in a clockwise direction to encourage positive results until the aloe butter is fully melted.

4. Add the candelilla wax. Again, stir the contents clockwise gently until wax is melted.

5. Add in the vitamin E oil, stir to combine, and turn off the heat.

6. Add in each essential oil. Stir clockwise once again and recite the following:

Soothe my hands and hydrate the skin.
Sacred calendula, let your magic begin.

7. Immediately pour into your jar and let cool. Ensure salve is completely cooled, about 45–60 minutes, before securing on the lid.

8. Apply as needed.

This salve should last at least 12 months when stored in a cool, dry place away from direct sunlight. The scents of the oils will fade over time, but if you notice they begin to smell rancid that will indicate it should be replaced.

Sunburn Soothing Mist

The sun is a life-giving star in this universe, and while it's lovely to embrace her transformational energies, stay too long and you will get burned. Associated with fire, the sun must be handled with care and respect. If you do happen to get a sunburn, you will want something on hand to help soothe the skin and fade the burn gently and efficiently.

Materials to Gather

- ½ teaspoon vegetable glycerin
- 4-ounce dark glass spray bottle
- 10 drops lemongrass essential oil
- 5 drops basil essential oil
- 5 drops lavender essential oil
- 4 teaspoons witch hazel
- 2 tablespoons eucalyptus floral water
- ¼ cup aloe vera juice

Steps to Take

1. Cleanse your workspace and gather your ingredients.

2. Ease your mind from any outside noise. Focus your energy on the healing powers of your ingredients. Visualize your sunburn feeling soothed, gently healing, and fading away. Hold this vision in your mind as you go through the mixing process.

3. Use a funnel to add the vegetable glycerin to the bottle.

4. Add in the essential oils.

5. Add the witch hazel, floral water, and aloe vera juice and place the cap on the bottle.

6. Shake the bottle and recite the following:

> Sunburn be soothed and fully healed.
> Let healthy skin be revealed.
> Renewed, revived, and free from pain.
> Calm and fresh like soft summer rain.

7. Your soothing mist is ready to use. Shake prior to each use. Apply as often as needed to soothe and relieve the skin. You may wish to recite the following affirmation each time you use your spray: "My sunburn has healed and faded away."

Rosemary Lemon Cuticle Oil

Cuticle oil is a moisturizer for your nails that nourishes, protects, and stimulates growth, but conventional ones are laden with harmful chemicals. Your hands are a critical component in your witchcraft practice and should be shown proper care. Nail issues can also be attributed to nutrition deficiencies, so while you're cleaning up your diet, use this cuticle oil each day to help achieve strong and healthy nails.

Materials to Gather

- 1-ounce dark glass dropper bottle
- 6 drops rosemary essential oil
- 4 drops lemon essential oil
- ¼ teaspoon vitamin E oil
- 4 teaspoons jojoba oil
- 2 teaspoons avocado oil

Steps to Take

1. Cleanse your workspace and gather your ingredients. Relax you mind and focus on the appreciation you have for your hands and nails. They do so much for you each day and should be shown some extra love and care.

2. Add the essential oils one at a time into your glass bottle.

3. Use a funnel to add in the vitamin E oil, jojoba oil, and avocado oil.

4. Secure the top on the bottle and shake for 30 seconds. Say:

Lemon and rosemary, nourish my nails.
Hydration and strength shall be unveiled.

5. To use, place a small drop on your cuticles one at a time and massage into the nail. Apply at least once per day; however, the more you apply, the better your results will be. Shake prior to each use.

Hair Rinse for Revitalization

Hair has been known as a common ingredient in various witchcraft practices for a very long time and is still used by some today. It's strong associations with power and strength make it easy to understand why. This rinse can help you achieve soft, smooth, and shiny tresses with the magical hair-healing abilities of nettle, chamomile, and marshmallow root.

Materials to Gather

- 3 cups water
- 1 tablespoon dried nettle
- 1 tablespoon dried chamomile
- 1 tablespoon dried marshmallow root

Steps to Take

1. Cleanse your workspace and gather your ingredients. Focus your thoughts toward your hair and making it strong and healthy.

2. Fill a medium pot with the water.

3. Add in the herbs one at a time. Recite the following as you do:

> *Sacred nettle, bring shine.*
> *Sacred chamomile, bring strength.*
> *Sacred marshmallow, bring growth.*

4. Turn the heat to high and bring to a boil. Reduce the heat to low, cover, and let simmer 10–20 minutes. Envision your hair looking shiny, healthy, and radiant.

5. Remove from heat and strain the liquid into your container of choice. Your rinse is ready! The rinse will keep in the refrigerator about 1 week.

6. Depending on how much hair you have, you will want to use ¼–1 cup of the rinse each time. You can use as often as you like, from every day to just once per week. To use the rinse, pour it onto your hair slowly so that it is not lost down the drain. Massage it into your scalp and tresses and let it sit 5 minutes before rinsing. While massaging, you may recite the following:

My hair will shine and sparkle bright.
Nourished and smooth from morning to night.
Healthy and strong for all to see.
As my will, so mote it be.

The herbal remedies included here are all most easily made in your kitchen for easy cleanup and access to ingredients. And be sure to always physically cleanse your space prior to beginning to avoid any contamination of your final product.

What makes tea magical? Thousands of cups of tea are brewed every day, but they aren't all creating magic; some are simply just delicious and soothing. What brings in the magical aspect is the plant's individual properties, and very importantly, the intentions and energy you hold while brewing.

Teas are simple infusions and one of the easiest and safest ways to reap the benefits of herbs. They're incredibly versatile and fun to create, and they can be used for spiritual and practical applications. The best herbs to use for teas are those that are pleasant and mild tasting, have high nutritional value, or require a high dosage to be effective. Drinking a cup of tea will provide your body with many physical benefits as well as the energetic properties held within the plant matter.

The following preparation method will enable you to craft a tea and infuse it with your magic and intentions. The six tea blends that follow will be prepared in the same way. For each recipe, you will use about 1 teaspoon of dried herb per 1 cup of water. If using fresh herbs, you may use 2 teaspoons per 1 cup of water.

Steps to Take

1. Choose your ingredients and set your intentions. Make them extremely specific and clear in your mind for each type of tea.

2. Fill your pot or kettle with water and bring to a boil.

3. Add your loose herbs into a tea ball, teapot, or directly into your cup. As you are adding your herbs, visualize the tea working its magic within yourself. If your intention is to promote good digestion, imagine the tea moving down through your digestive system, assisting everything to run smoothly and efficiently. Imagine yourself free from any digestive discomfort, feeling relaxed and strong.

4. Once your water is boiled, pour it over the herbs and let your blend steep for 10–15 minutes. The longer you steep, the stronger the infusion. For tougher parts of a plant such as roots and bark, you will want to add the herbs directly into the pot with your water, bring water to a boil, simmer for 15–20 minutes, then strain; this type of tea is considered a decoction as opposed to an infusion.

5. If necessary remove your tea ball, focus your gaze on your tea, and recite the following:

Blessed herbs, release your magic; blessed herbs, heal me well. I give thanks for your aid and help with this spell.

6. While you drink, envision the tea doing its healing work. Drink with intention and gratitude. You may add additional spells or chants to match each purpose if you wish.

When using dried or fresh herbs for teas, ensure that they are culinary grade, and organic is best, if possible.

Cinnamon Cardamom Blend to Balance Blood Sugar

Magically, these herbs both contain strong energies, including love, balance, and success. For physical benefits, they contain properties that may aid in the regulation of blood sugar in the body. Cinnamon slows the release of insulin into the bloodstream, causing blood sugar levels to rise more slowly after a meal, and cardamom may regulate glucose metabolism in the body.

When you're using cinnamon, it's important to use Ceylon cinnamon, known as "true cinnamon," and not the cassia varieties. Large amounts of cassia cinnamon can have adverse side effects, and you would need twice as much to get the same health benefits as with Ceylon.

Materials to Gather

- 1⅓ cups boiling water
- 2 cardamom pods
- 1 teaspoon ground Ceylon cinnamon or 1 crushed stick

This blend is also delicious with a touch of frothed or warmed non-dairy milk.

Carob Lavender Blend to Banish Cravings

This is a delightful blend that can substitute as a sweet treat and ease those sugar cravings. Carob is low in fat, contains antioxidants, and is naturally sweet, making it a great substitute for chocolate. Lavender promotes happiness and is a wonderfully complementary flavor to the carob, which carries properties of love, health, and prosperity.

Materials to Gather

- ½ cup boiling water
- ½ cup nondairy milk
- 1 teaspoon carob powder
- ½ teaspoon dried lavender buds
- ½ teaspoon pure maple syrup (optional)

If you wish to add maple syrup, you may add it in once the tea has steeped.

Lemon Peppermint Blend for Improved Digestion

This is an effective digestive tea that will perk you up at the same time. Peppermint relaxes the muscles in the digestive tract, making for a smoother digestive process, while lemon is thought to be a digestive stimulant and aids in getting your system moving. This combo will provide you with uplifting and renewed energies, making it optimal for mornings or after meals.

Materials to Gather

- 1 cup boiling water
- 1 teaspoon dried peppermint
- Juice from 1–2 lemon wedges

For the lemon wedges, you may squeeze the juice and then drop the wedges directly in your cup, or just squeeze the juice and discard the wedges.

Nettle Dandelion Blend for Liver Detox

Nettle and dandelion are well known for their powerful detox effects on the body. Dandelion helps to detox your liver, and nettle supports functions of the liver and kidneys. Both of these herbs also contain energetic healing properties, making them a wonderful combo for physical and energetic healing within the body. This tea will help you feel cleansed, lighter, and happier on the inside.

Materials to Gather

- 1 cup boiling water
- ½ teaspoon dried nettle
- ½ teaspoon dried dandelion
- Juice from 1 lemon wedge

Hibiscus Blend to Boost Metabolism

The herbs here all have positive effects on metabolism. Your metabolism consists of the complex chemical processes that allow your body to properly function. The faster your metabolism, the more energy your body will require to make these processes happen. A healthy metabolism provides more energy and better overall functioning throughout your body's systems. Magically, this tea contains loving, uplifting, and positive energies that will greatly benefit your spirit and motivation levels.

Materials to Gather

- 1½ cups boiling water
- ½ teaspoon dried hibiscus
- ½ teaspoon dried lemongrass
- ½ teaspoon dried peppermint

Lemon Balm Blend to Banish Brain Fog

Lemon balm is a delicious herb that promotes enhanced cognitive function. It's also a calming herb, and when you're calm it's much easier to concentrate and focus the mind. Oranges, not to be confused with sweet orange essential oil, also provides better brain function and alertness in the body. Magically, the pair can promote happiness, renewed energies, and positivity—all elements that encourage a healthy brain and mind.

Materials to Gather

- 1 cup boiling water
- 1 teaspoon dried lemon balm
- Juice from 1 orange wedge

Take used lemon and orange wedges from your teas and save them in the refrigerator. You can use them later to craft simmer pots for joy, positivity, and cleansing.

PHYSICAL WELLNESS JOURNAL PROMPTS AND AFFIRMATIONS

The following journal prompts and affirmations will help to keep your mind clear on what you would like to get out of this new magical wellness path in terms of your physical self. They can help to solidify your intentions and enable you to stay on track throughout your new journey.

Journal Prompts for Physical Wellness

1. What is one new habit you will adopt to benefit your physical wellness?

2. What three symptoms do you experience regularly that you would like to address?

3. What form of movement gets you excited to get up in the morning?

4. What will you include in your morning routine? Bedtime routine?

5. What are the five words you would like to use to describe your physical wellness?

Daily Affirmations for Physical Wellness

- I am healthy; I am strong.
- I am vibrant and thriving.
- My body is working efficiently and smoothly each day.

- My body is energetic and rested.
- My body is my sacred vessel and I will honor it.

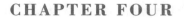

CHAPTER FOUR

Magic for Mental and Emotional Wellness

Your witchcraft practice plays a pivotal role in your overall mental health. Incorporating magic into your life will lower stress, boost confidence, provide you with a stronger sense of self, and gift you with a sense of mindfulness within yourself and your surroundings. It enriches your life and your mental well-being in magical and mystical ways if you let it.

Your mind is an enchanting and fascinating place. It's the place where your magic is first established. The thoughts and emotions that prompt you to perform a spell or ritual are created there, and the outcome of your magical workings is reliant on the mind's focus, intent, and will to reach the desired goal. You must care for and acknowledge your thoughts and emotions to produce the most effective outcomes in your witchcraft practice and in order to achieve your best personal state of wellness.

Everything that you do and accomplish on this magical wellness journey will begin in your mind. Your mind is what guides you to make decisions, be motivated, dream, and learn. You can use this incredible power and knowledge to shape your life into something magical and amazing, but you must take the time to tend to it, nurture it, and keep it engaged.

Mental health and wellness are often overlooked or not taken as seriously as the health and wellness of the physical body, but this is a very sad oversight. The processes inside the mind directly affect chemical reactions in the body as well as how open we are to spirit and the greater universe around us. An unhealthy mind can manifest in many different illnesses and energy blocks in the physical body. In this chapter, we will discuss beating negative self-talk, moving toward self-acceptance, dealing with stress and anxiety, healing your emotional self, and boosting happy hormones in the body.

Self-acceptance is being okay with who you are, embracing yourself with all of your beautiful flaws as well as your gifts. This doesn't mean you don't want to become a better version of yourself, but it does mean each day you accept where you're at and are comfortable being in that space.

Without self-acceptance, your mental health suffers and anxiety, depression, addiction, and other health concerns can begin to creep in. You must love yourself and believe that you are worth loving in order to thrive. We tend to direct a lot of negativity toward ourselves for not being stronger, better, smarter, more attractive, or any number of other traits. What if you could accept all of the things about yourself and realize that you already are strong, smart, and exquisite in your own individual ways?

If you allow your mind to be free from things that do not serve it well, such as negative self-talk, that is when your personal energies will be able to soar. Your mind will become unburdened and open to create powerful change in all areas of your life. Those negative aspects take up space that would be better allotted to making yourself more confident and prosperous, or channeled toward reaching new heights in your witchcraft practice.

Coming into yourself, knowing your true self, and loving every bit of that self is when your wellness and your magic will both begin to flourish and your magical wellness path will become that much clearer.

Ritual to Banish Negative Thought Patterns

Negative self-talk is truly a plague that prohibits you from experiencing so much of what life has to offer. Perfection is an illusion that should be dismantled and set on fire, for when you decide to burn it down, you will finally be able to emerge like a luminous moth rising out of its cocoon into your most powerful state as you were always meant to do. The following ritual will help you to release these negative thought patterns brought on by the human quest for perfection.

Materials to Gather

- 1 black candle for releasing negativity
- 3 black tourmaline stones for cleansing, grounding, and positivity
- Piece of paper and a pen
- Cauldron or firesafe dish
- Small dish of salt
- 1 stick sandalwood incense for banishing and healing

Steps to Take

1. Cleanse, ground, and center as needed.

2. Clear your mind and sit comfortably in your space. Take three deeps breaths and relax your shoulders. Try to bring your mind to a place of calm.

3. Light your candle and place the black tourmaline stones in a circle around it, one each to represent cleansing, grounding, and positivity.

4. Focus your mind toward any negative thoughts you have been having recently. What thoughts come up all of the time that have no positive purpose and you would like to be rid of?

5. After thinking on these for a minute, take your pen and paper and write down anything you can think of that does not serve you in your life or on your magical wellness journey. These thoughts are not true; they are your inner critic trying to hold you back and have you believe that you will never be good enough. You are better and stronger than these thoughts, and it's time to let them go.

6. Once you have everything written down, tear the piece of paper up as many times as feels good. With every rip of the paper, imagine these thoughts being expelled from your mind. These thoughts do not deserve your energy.

7. Place the torn paper into your cauldron or firesafe dish and sprinkle the pieces with the salt. Recite the following:

Negative thoughts, I let you go.
Leave my mind and let things flow.
Release the dark and embrace the light.
Permission is granted to leave my sight.

8. Now take your incense stick and light the end. Before the flame goes out, light the paper in your cauldron or firesafe dish and watch your negativity being burned away into nothingness.

9. Focus on the flame and allow your mind to feel free, light, and ready to welcome in new positive energy and thought patterns.

10. If safe to do so, allow the papers, candle, and incense to burn down on their own. Do not leave unattended.

Ylang-Ylang Salt Bath to Ignite Self-Confidence

There will be days when your confidence is lacking and you are not feeling like your most vibrant self. Hopefully, you will have fewer of them as you move along this magical wellness journey, but sometimes you may need a little confidence boost, and indulging in a relaxing ritual bath may be just the thing.

Materials to Gather

- 1 yellow candle for confidence and charm
- 1 stick lemon balm incense for confidence and success
- ½ cup Himalayan pink salt for love and self-esteem
- ½ cup pink rose petals for self-love and rebirth
- 6 drops ylang-ylang essential oil for confidence and happiness
- 3 drops patchouli essential oil for growth and beauty

Steps to Take

1. Cleanse, ground, and center as needed.

2. Relax your mind while preparing your bathroom for your ritual. Take your time to set up your materials, lay out something that makes you feel good to put on afterward, and add in any special touches you wish to include to help set the mood, such as music that makes you feel empowered or a glass of wine.

3. Once your space is prepared, light your candle and incense and begin to run your bath.

4. While the water is running, slowly add in your ingredients one at a time in the order they are listed. During this process, focus your mind on things you love about yourself: your favorite qualities, features, and talents that make you feel good and happy.

5. When the bathtub is sufficiently filled, turn the water off, gently step into the tub, and settle yourself comfortably. Take a few moments here to close your eyes and imagine your most amazing self walking down the street filled with confidence and positivity, or at work successfully completing all of your tasks with ease, or at your altar manifesting all of your greatest desires. You are capable of all these things and much more.

6. Make a commitment to always believe in yourself and your abilities. You can achieve anything you set your mind to. Recite the following:

> Intelligent and strong, I've found my place.
> Timeless beauty and filled with grace.
> Worthy and magic, I can finally see.
> As my will, so mote it be.

7. Spend as much time as you like relaxing in this space and frame of mind. Once finished you may extinguish your incense and candle or allow them to burn down fully if safe to do so.

-⟨⟨⟨-

Mirror Spell for Self-Acceptance

Mirrors have long been a source of magic—mystical gateways and portals to other realms. In this practice, we will be using the mirror as a tool toward self-acceptance. Instead of looking into the mirror and judging yourself, you will use it to allow yourself to be seen and loved. Repeat this ritual as often as you feel it's needed. You could even complete a mini version of this each day as part of your morning routine.

Materials to Gather

- Mirror
- 2 purple candles for wisdom, healing, and understanding your true self

Steps to Take

1. Begin by cleansing your mirror of any dust, fingerprints, or old lingering energies. You may consider wiping the mirror down with a cloth and then cleansing the energies with a purification incense such as lemon balm or chamomile. Now bring yourself into a balanced and positive frame of mind.

2. Wash your face so that it is free from any makeup or mask you may have been wearing. You want to see yourself in all of your natural and magical glory.

3. Set your candles on either side of the mirror and light them.

4. Now sit comfortably, clear your mind, and take the next 5 minutes to stare at yourself in the mirror. Really look at your features and appreciate them, take a moment to tell yourself five of your best personal qualities, and think of three things you consider your flaws that you have always tried to change. Hold in your mind these special traits that are unique to you, the positive ones and the presumed flaws. Stare into your eyes and recite the following:

> *Eyes wide open, ripe and raw.*
> *I accept myself through every flaw.*
> *Unique and beautiful, from stars to sea.*
> *Completely whole, and perfectly me.*

5. Now imagine the frame of your mirror illuminating in a brilliant purple light. Trace a heart in the center of the mirror with your finger and say, "So mote it be." You may now extinguish your flames.

Mirrors have long been thought to be a powerful magical tool. They have been used to heal, to uncover truth, in scrying, as well as for revisiting past lives and glamour magic. Experiment with different positive ways of adding mirror magic into your practice. Allow yourself to gaze, enchant, and fully see yourself without judgement.

Self-Love Spell Jar

A huge component of transforming into your most magical self is getting to a calm place where you know that you have pure and unconditional love for yourself. Without self-love, your mind can become overrun with doubt, fear, and anxiety. The following spell jar will help serve as a reminder that you are worthy of love and deserve to feel it every day.

Materials to Gather

- Small Mason jar with lid
- 1 pink candle for self-esteem and love
- 1 white candle for cleansing and renewal
- 3 tablespoons dried lemon balm for love, confidence, and happiness
- 1 amethyst stone for love
- 1 lapis lazuli stone for confidence
- 1 moonstone for rebirth
- 3 drops bergamot essential oil for confidence and success
- 1 long pink ribbon for love and tranquility

Steps to Take

1. Cleanse, ground, and center as needed.

2. Clear your mind and prepare your space.

3. Sit comfortably and set your Mason jar in the middle of your space with one candle on either side.

4. Light your candles. Focus on you in this moment. Work on feeling positive and loving emotions toward yourself. Let them fill you up from deep inside your core. Imagine these feelings as pink sparkles swirling in your center, then branching out to reach every inch of you, down to your toes, out to your fingertips, and to the top of your head.

5. Add the lemon balm into your jar, then the crystals, and then the essential oil. While filling your jar, keep the image of the pink

sparkles swirling within, spreading love through every inch of yourself.

6. Lastly, tie the ends of the pink ribbon together so that it forms a circle. This circle represents the continuous circle of love you feel for yourself, secure and unbreakable. Place the ribbon inside the jar and close the lid.

7. Place both hands above the jar, close your eyes, and recite the following three times:

I accept myself and love myself unconditionally.

8. You may now extinguish your flames and place the jar in an area where you will regularly see it as a reminder of this commitment to yourself.

Simmer Pot for Mental Strength

This simmer pot is perfect to brew in the morning on a day that you know will require you to stay mentally strong and focused. A big day at work, a difficult conversation, or a particularly challenging ritual are all times when this simmer pot would be good to have on hand.

Materials to Gather

- Small pot filled with water
- 1 tablespoon dried basil for strength
- 1 tablespoon dried sage for mental clarity
- 4 apple slices for success
- 3 lime slices for strength and calm

Steps to Take

1. Cleanse, ground, and center as needed.

2. Gather your ingredients and relax your mind. Direct your focus to feeling a strong sense of self and confidence in your mind's eye. Visualize yourself moving throughout your day with courage and assurance.

3. Place your pot with water on the stove over medium-high heat.

4. Add in the ingredients one at a time. While adding in each ingredient, focus on the properties it carries.

5. Once the ingredients are added, stir the contents with a wooden spoon clockwise three times to promote positivity and good fortune.

6. Allow the pot to come to a boil. Keep focus on your intentions during this time.

7. Once the water is boiling, turn the heat down to low and let simmer. Recite the following:

> I reach within to search and find.
> May these gifts from the earth bring strength of mind.
> Courage and confidence flow through me.
> This is my will, so mote it be.

8. Let the pot simmer as you prepare for your day but be careful not to let it boil dry. Simply add more water if it gets low.

You may also start this process 1 or 2 days before the big day for added effectiveness. The ingredients are fine to be reboiled, and repeating the process will amplify your spell and build your strength up over these few days. You may compost (if applicable) the ingredients once your work is complete.

When certain emotions arise from trauma or loss, they can be extremely difficult to heal. This pain that you hang on to can cause many energy blockages in the body, leading to physical, mental, and spiritual symptoms manifesting.

Releasing emotional wounds from the past is integral for a healthy holistic self, and magic can be an incredibly therapeutic tool. Using your magic to assist with this can greatly increase your ability to let go of the pain and finally begin to heal. You may tend to push emotions down or aside and consider them dealt with, but true healing requires more work. When emotional scars are simply pushed to the side, they will fester and grow until they are fully acknowledged, accepted, and released.

Releasing painful emotions has many benefits to your health and well-being. Once you release these feelings, you may also begin to heal physical symptoms you've been experiencing, clear away mental blocks that have been hindering your magical practice, and reach an overall happier mental state. Healing takes time and dedication; simply performing a spell or ritual will not evaporate all the pain or negativity inside, but it's a start. With an optimistic mindset and some consistency, you will be on your way to healing fully and completely.

Ritual for Emotional Acceptance

Coming to a place of acceptance and acknowledgment of unpleasant memories will allow you to finally heal and free yourself from the emotions that have been holding you back from your own personal growth. This ritual can assist you in coming to terms with these emotions, enabling you to fully release them.

Materials to Gather

- 1 stick eucalyptus incense for personal growth
- Handful of dried rose petals or rosebuds for emotional healing
- Small glass jar with lid

Steps to Take

1. Cleanse, ground, and center as needed.

2. Seat yourself in a quiet space where you are comfortable, clear your mind, and light your incense.

3. Focus your thoughts on the emotions that have been dominating your heart and mind in recent days. Take a moment to sit with these emotions and acknowledge each of them, both positive and negative.

4. Fill your jar with the rose petals or rosebuds, placing them in one by one. Assign an emotion to each as you drop it in the jar. With each petal or rosebud, make a statement such as the following: "Frustration, I accept you," or "Pain, I accept you." They can also be positive emotions. Take time with this and don't leave any prominent emotions out of the jar.

5. Once your jar is filled, close the lid and recite the following:

Elements of me, within and without.
I accept and acknowledge, leaving no doubt.
These emotions no longer controlling me.
And as I choose, shall set them free.

6. By acknowledging your feelings, you are now ready to release any that are holding you back and to embrace the ones that are feeding you in a positive way. Allow your incense to burn down fully if safe to do so.

Emotional Cleansing Fire Ritual

The fire element is full of beautiful cleansing energies, and tapping in to these vibrations will assist you in letting go of painful and negative emotions in your mind. In this ritual, you will embrace fire and allow it to aid you in releasing emotions that are not serving you in a positive way.

Materials to Gather

- 1 white candle for cleansing
- Piece of paper and a pen
- Cauldron or firesafe dish

Steps to Take

1. Clear your mind and sit relaxed in your space.

2. Light your candle and focus your mind on the emotions you generally try to push to the side, such as fear, guilt, or shame. Bring these emotions to the surface and let yourself open up to fully let them in. Think about the instances in your life that caused them; however painful, these are your experiences and should be acknowledged. Allow yourself to feel vulnerable. Every experience has played a part in shaping you into the strong person you have become. Give acceptance to these experiences and the emotions they have produced within you. You must accept them before letting go.

3. Take your paper and pen and write down the top three to five emotions you are holding inside that you know in your heart must be released.

4. Hold the paper, use your candle to carefully light a corner on fire, and drop the paper into your cauldron or firesafe dish.

5. Stare into the flame in the cauldron or firesafe dish and feel your strength rising up and these negative emotions dissipating. With every breath you take, you are overcoming the emotions that have been holding you back from being your most magical and empowered self.

6. Recite the following:

I release my fear; I let it go.
Let my true strength bravely show.
No more buried pain, nothing but a memory.
I accept these emotions and boldly set them free.

7. Visualize the emotions you wrote down on your paper transforming into a bright white light illuminating up from your cauldron or firesafe dish. The transformative magic of the fire element is doing its work of shifting these negative emotions into positivity, strength, and courage. If safe to do so, allow the paper to burn out fully on its own. Allow your candle to burn down as well if you are able to. Thank the fire element for its aid. Your work is now complete.

Meditation for Emotional Healing

Meditation creates a sense of mindfulness, awareness, and recognition within yourself that is key for healing pain you may be holding in your mind and heart. This meditation will help you work on sitting with your emotions and allowing them to begin healing and fading away.

Materials to Gather

- 1 stick peppermint incense for healing and renewal

Steps to Take

1. Cleanse, ground, and center as needed.

2. Choose a quiet space where you will not be disturbed, relax your mind, and light your incense.

3. Sit comfortably and close your eyes. For about 60 seconds just focus on your breathing. Concentrate on making it slow, deep, and steady. Now focus for a moment on any negative emotions that have been plaguing you. Imagine each of these emotions as a crack in your mind.

4. Now in the center of your forehead imagine a glowing blue light in the shape of a diamond. Visualize this light pushing inward through your forehead and reaching toward the very edges of your mind. As it travels and spreads its light, imagine the blue healing light closing up each of the cracks as it passes over them. Once all the cracks have been sealed, imagine your mind surrounded by this luminous, healing blue light and recite the following in your mind:

*Cracks now sealed, my mind
fully formed.
Refreshed, renewed, it's weath-
ered this storm.*

5. Stay in your meditation, holding the image of your mind illuminating in the healing blue light,

and repeat the deep breathing for 60 seconds as you did in the beginning. Once finished, open your eyes and say, "So mote it be." Extinguish your incense or allow it to burn down fully if safe to do so.

Full Moon Ritual to Release Fear

Fear is an emotion that keeps you safe but can also hold you back from experiencing life to the fullest. Healthy fear is crucial for your survival, while unhealthy fear is something created in your mind that has no real bearing in reality. This type of fear is what keeps you in your comfort zone and should be overcome. The full moon is an opportune time to perform this type of banishing magic.

Materials to Gather

- 1 black candle
- 1 red candle
- 1 white candle
- Pin or ritual knife

Steps to Take

1. Cleanse, ground, and center as needed.

2. Gather your materials and clear your mind. Try and bring yourself into a centered state. Conjure within yourself feelings of determination, strength, and focus.

Know that you are stronger than your fear, and bring yourself into this frame of mind.

3. Take your black candle and carve "I release my fear" into it with your pin or knife. It doesn't have to be pretty or neat; just carve it in as best you can. Once it is carved, say the words aloud, place the candle in the center of your space, and light it.

4. Next, take your red candle and carve the word "strength" into it, set it slightly forward and to the side of your black candle, and light it. Say, "I am strong."

5. Lastly, take your white candle and carve the word "renewal" into it, set it in line with your red candle on the other side of the black one, light it, and say, "I am renewed."

6. At this point your candles should all be lit and form a triangle with the black one positioned in the center at the top. Close your eyes, lift both of your arms overhead with your palms pointing toward the sky. Recite the following (out loud is best, so that the universe hears you)

> *I call upon the full moon light.*
> *Take this darkness and make it right.*
> *I release my fear and stand here strong.*
> *Shadow within be fully gone.*

7. Keep your eyes closed and imagine your fear swirling up through your body like a cloud of black smoke, traveling out through your fingertips and disappearing into the night sky.

8. Open your eyes, give thanks to the full moon for her energy and strength. If possible, allow your candles to burn down at least past the words you carved into them, signifying the completion of your spell. If you know you won't have too much time, you may carve the words closer to the top of the candle so they won't need as much time to burn.

The energy of a full moon can be incredibly beneficial to your rituals and spell work. Pay attention to the moon's phases so that you may incorporate more of its energy into your practice. The full moon is particularly good for healing, prosperity, love, wisdom, and divination work. Some witches also choose to simply channel this energy into whatever their most important magical work may be at the time.

Memory Ritual to Boost Happiness

Memories can trigger all sorts of emotions within you, and your senses can trigger different types of memories. For this ritual, you are going to call on the strength of your happiest memories as a reminder to yourself that in dark times there are always places of light to draw from.

Materials to Gather

- Piece of paper and a pen
- 1 pink candle

Steps to Take

1. Cleanse, ground, and center as needed.

2. Sit comfortably, clear your mind, and light your candle. Let your troubles gently melt away. It is not time for them right now.

3. Take your paper and pen and write down ten memories you have that fill your heart with happiness and joy. Take your time and allow yourself to fully remember each one as you work through the ten. It can be a memory of the simplest thing as long as it brought happiness to your heart. Re-create the memory in your mind with the feelings, the sights, and the sounds that went with it.

4. Once you are done with all ten, fold the paper into three and hold it to your heart. Recite the following:

*Memories of joy stay with me.
Never forgotten and always seen.
Allow them to bring love to my heart.
In my mind they shall never part.*

5. You may now extinguish your flame. Take your paper and place it on your altar, inside a special box, or in a drawer. Revisit this list on days when things are feeling tough as a reminder of these special moments in your life that have made you laugh, smile, and feel joy. Feel free to also add to the list if a new special moment happens that you think should be included.

Spell Sachet to Overcome Addiction

Whether it's cigarettes, alcohol, food, or any other substance, it takes an incredible amount of resilience and strength to push through the haze of addiction and get to a place of clarity. You may carry this sachet in your bag or on your person and store in a prominent place to help give you the strength to persevere.

Materials to Gather

- 1 stick lemon balm incense for success
- 1 tablespoon dried peppermint for renewal
- 1 tablespoon dried hibiscus for healing
- 1 tablespoon dried basil for hope
- Mortar and pestle
- Small gold pouch for positivity and strength to overcome addiction
- 1 amethyst stone for new beginnings
- 1 carnelian stone for motivation
- 1 citrine stone for confidence
- 3 drops patchouli essential oil for growth

Steps to Take

1. Cleanse, ground, and center as needed.

2. Clear your mind and prepare your space. Focus your thoughts on your addiction and how you will feel once you overcome it. What will your days look like? What emotions will fill you up deep inside at your core? Imagine what things will be like once the addiction is a thing of the past and you have moved on to a new place in your life.

3. Sit comfortably to promote a sense of calm, and light your incense.

4. Clear your head and focus your mind on feelings of determination, motivation, strength, and resilience, all things that you are and that you have inside yourself.

5. Add in each herb individually to your mortar and begin blending them together. Visualize the energy of determination surrounding your entire body in a beautiful golden hue, infusing you with this powerful emotion and strong sense of self. You can do this. Believe that this is the time for change.

6. Once the herbs are blended, pour them into your pouch and tie it up. Hold the pouch to your heart and recite these lines:

The time has come to be well.
Addiction, be released with this spell.
My mind unchained, strong, and free.
As my will, so mote it be.

7. Add the three crystals and then the essential oil to the pouch. Tie up the pouch, hold it in your hands, close your eyes, and state with undisputed resolve: "I believe in me." Allow your incense to burn down fully.

It's a good idea to keep this sachet with you or close by you, especially when you are first beginning this particular journey. This is especially important in situations or at times when you know you may need to overcome temptation.

Sunrise Ritual for Renewal

This magical time of day when the sun is awakening from the night's slumber to shine and provide strength and warmth to the earth is a time that represents renewal and change. Your mind, like your body and spirit, will benefit from an occasional reset. This sunrise ritual will help you channel this vibrant energy to refresh and rejuvenate your mind.

Materials to Gather

- 1 white ribbon for cleansing
- 1 gold ribbon for connection to the sun
- 1 amethyst stone for new beginnings
- 1 peridot stone for transformation

Steps to Take

1. Cleanse, ground, and center as needed.

2. Find a tranquil space outside on a sunny day. If necessary, this can also be performed indoors

in front of a sunny window, but it's important for the sun to be illuminating your skin, igniting transformation and renewal within your mind and body.

3. Sit comfortably and tie your ribbons around your wrists, one on each.

4. Take your stones, one in each hand, and hold them for the duration of your ritual.

5. Close your eyes and clear your mind of any outside noise and distractions. Feel the sunshine on your skin providing vitality and transformational energies.

6. Visualize a brilliant gold sparkling light taking shape in the center of your mind. Imagine this light spreading out to the farthest reaches of your mind and clearing out any stressors or negativities that may be dwelling there. Take your time and keep this visualization until you imagine your entire mind is glowing bright and strong, filled with this gold sparkling light energy.

7. Either out loud or in your mind recite the following:

Clear this space and ease my mind.
Magic within I shall find.
Make room for the new and release the old.
What enters now shines like gold.

8. Open your eyes and spend some time basking in the beautiful energies of the sun in this renewed, joyful, and cleansed frame of mind.

To overcome an addiction is a long and arduous road. Magic, like the sachet we've crafted here, is meant to be but a tool to aid you on the path toward healing and persevering. It should never be relied upon as an easy fix or cure-all method, nor should it take the place of advice and treatment from a medical professional.

Stress and anxiety wreak havoc on the body, mind, and spirit. Since the mind is where the thoughts that ignite these stressful reactions are formed, if you control your thoughts, you control your stress and anxiety levels in the body. Stress and anxiety are the body's responses to danger; however, most of the times when you experience these things there is no real danger present. You may be feeling concern about something that has happened or something that hasn't yet happened.

Holding on to stress in the body causes an erratic flow in energy that contributes to heart disease, obesity, diabetes, depression, and unreliable magical work. This can lead to spells and rituals that either don't amount to much or don't turn out the way you had planned. Your energy when performing magic should be centred, balanced, and calm so that it may be directed and channeled in the manner of your intentions. The following practices can help to ease your mind when stress, anxiety, and worry arise.

Five-Minute Ritual for Easing Anxiety

This ritual is short and sweet. It's meant to be utilized when you are suffering from a particularly bad, or unexpected, episode of anxiety in order to ease your mind and release the feelings of stress. You may repeat the ritual as often as needed or make it a daily practice to help keep anxiety at bay.

Materials to Gather

- 1 white candle

Steps to Take

1. Cleanse, ground, and center as needed.

2. Sit comfortably and light your candle.

3. Relax your shoulders and stare into your flame. Focus on completing long, deep breaths. You want to open up your lungs and allow them to be filled with air. Count to four on your inhale and

again to four on the exhale. Don't rush. Imagine your lungs filling up with a soothing iridescent light with every inhale you take, and on each exhale imagine the anxiety being released from the body and dissipating into nothingness.

4. Continue in this state and focusing on your flame for about 4 minutes. When the time is through, place both hands, one on top of the other, in the center of your chest and close your eyes. Say, "I call on my inner strength and inner magic as a witch to release these feelings of anxiety from my heart, mind, and spirit. They hold no power or control over me."

5. Open your eyes, snuff out your flame, and say, "And so it shall be."

Spell Jar to Alleviate Worry

Excessive worry will negatively impact your health and magical work. It's also something only you can control. You must trust in yourself and in the universe that all will be well while also making practical decisions around the situation and utilizing your magic to shift the energies more favorably to your desired outcome. The following ritual will help you to accept situations as they are and release the worry you're feeling.

Materials to Gather

- Small Mason jar with lid
- 1 blue candle for peace and insight
- 1 orange candle for encouragement and good luck
- 3 tablespoons dried yarrow for relaxation, calm, and happiness
- 1 tiger's eye stone for balance
- 1 hematite stone for banishing
- 1 citrine stone for optimism
- 3 drops tea tree essential oil for strength and peace
- 1 blue ribbon

Steps to Take

1. Cleanse, ground, and center as needed.

2. Clear your mind and gather your ingredients.

3. Sit comfortably and set your Mason jar in the middle of your space with one candle on either side.

4. Light your candles. Focus on releasing feelings of worry. Trust in your heart all will be well and

you have already done everything to have the situation turn out favorably. Accept the feelings of worry, the true reason for them, and then let them go. Feel that sense of worry you are holding in your center, acknowledge it, and allow it to shift toward feelings of faith, hope, and assurance.

5. Add the yarrow into the jar, then your crystals and essential oil. While filling your jar, focus on these renewed feelings of assurance that things will work out. Truly believe them and feel them in your heart, head, and center.

6. Lastly, tie the ends of your blue ribbon together so that it forms a circle. This circle represents the unbroken trust you have in yourself, in the elements, and in the universe. Place the ribbon in your jar and secure the lid.

7. Place both hands above the jar, close your eyes, and recite the following three times:

I release my worries and replace them with strength, resilience, and calm.

8. You may now extinguish your flames and place the jar in an area where you will regularly see it as a reminder to remain calm, not worry about things you cannot change, and embrace the ever-present moments in life.

Candle Ritual for Combating Stress

Stress is a damaging feeling to hold on to and will create energy within your body that can contribute to an impaired immune system, which can in turn lead to illness. It will also create blockages that will be hard to overcome within your magical practice. This ritual is best done during the waning phase of the moon, which is a perfect time for spells related to banishing. Alternatively, you could perform it on a Sunday or Monday as these days being ruled by the Sun and the Moon have strong healing energies.

Materials to Gather

- 1–2 drops ylang-ylang essential oil (properly diluted) for confidence and calm
- 1 red candle for strength and vitality

Steps to Take

1. Cleanse, ground, and center as needed.

2. Sit comfortably in your space, place a drop or two of the ylang-ylang essential oil on your index finger, and anoint your candle with it. Run your finger up the sides and around the center until you are satisfied. Be sure to use only a small amount of oil.

3. Now light your candle and close your eyes. Visualize yourself as being stress-free. What would your days look like if you were no longer dealing with stress in the body? How much more joy and appreciation would you experience? Stay in this visualization of your most carefree and relaxed self for at least 5 minutes. Let your mind wander and imagine what it would be like to be free from these unsettling energies within yourself.

4. Once you finish, open your eyes and recite the following:

> Stress, be gone; I've no place for you.
> Energies relaxed my whole self through.
> Calm and centred is my mind.
> Peace within I shall find.

5. Give thanks, say, "So it shall be done," and extinguish your flame.

Calming Ritual Salt Bath

There is hardly a more relaxing activity than a soothing bath to bring your mind back to a place of peace and calm. This ritual will draw on the healing powers of the salts and calming energies of the oils to ease the mind and nervous system back into a more balanced state.

Materials to Gather

- 1 blue candle for calm and insight
- 1 stick sandalwood incense for peace
- 1 cup Dead Sea salts (or Epsom salts) for cleansing and healing
- 6 drops neroli essential oil for relaxation and joy
- 3 drops lavender essential oil for balance and calm

Steps to Take

1. Cleanse, ground, and center as needed.

2. Relax your mind and set up your materials in your space. Take this time to center yourself, focus your energy, and forget about any stresses from the day.

3. Once your space is prepared, light your candle and incense and begin to run your bath.

4. While your water is running, slowly add in your ingredients one at a time in the order they are listed. During this process, focus on slowing your breathing, take long deep breaths, close your eyes, relax your shoulders, and ease your mind.

5. When the bathtub is sufficiently filled, turn the water off, gently step into the tub, and settle yourself comfortably. Take a few moments here to close your eyes and imagine a beautiful green thread of light spiraling in your center and then working its way out to the rest of your body evenly and slowly. Visualize this thread bringing balance to your mind and allowing your whole self to feel relaxed and at ease. You are grounded and without stress.

6. Relax into this sense of peace and calm. Your anxieties and stress are not in control of you.

You are in control of you. Recite the following:

> *Balance and peace deep within.*
> *Let this calming spell begin.*
> *I break the chains holding me.*
> *This is my will, so mote it be.*

Relaxation Meditation with Crystals

The healing energies of crystals can be wonderful additions to your meditation practice. The crystals used in the following ritual will help to release tension from the mind, allowing it to become calm and relaxed.

Materials to Gather

- 1 stick chamomile incense to ease anxiety and uplift the mind
- 1 amethyst stone to encourage relaxation and calm
- 1 clear quartz stone for clarity
- 1 lepidolite stone to ease anxiety

Steps to Take

1. Cleanse, ground, and center as needed.

2. Choose a space where you can lie down and will not be disturbed.

3. Light your incense and then lie down comfortably.

4. Place your amethyst crystal in the center of your forehead, allowing it to work its magic by clearing away any energy blocks that may be occurring in this area. This will help to calm the mind and open up the flow of energy through this space.

5. Now take the clear quartz and lepidolite and hold one in each hand with your palms closed.

6. Close your eyes and allow your muscles to relax; feel yourself sinking into your space and releasing any tension you may be holding. Focus on your breath for a moment. Feel the deep inhale and release on the exhale. Imagine with each exhale you are releasing any stresses or worries from your mind, and each inhale is

7. Spend as much time as you are able to relaxing in this space. Focus your mind on things that make you feel happy, calm, and at peace. Once finished, you may extinguish your flame and incense.

welcoming in positivity and light. With each breath, you are entering a more relaxed and centered state.

7. Stay in this place for at least 5 minutes, though you can stay as long as you would like or are able to. Focus on only your breath and letting go of stressful thoughts that may be plaguing your mind. If you lose focus, don't despair; just take a breath and bring yourself back to this place.

8. Once you feel your time is complete, open your eyes and say, "I am relaxed and calm. The tensions of my day do not control me." Take one final breath, thank the crystals for their service, and rise from your space. If it hasn't yet, allow your incense to burn down fully.

Sunset Ritual to Help Ease Symptoms of Depression

As the sun sets on the horizon, it presents effective energies for releasing negative thoughts and emotional states such as depression, anxiety, and worry. This ritual will call on these energies to help provide you with a path of light to follow when days seem their darkest and it's hard to see past them to brighter days.

Materials to Gather

- 1 stick lemon balm incense for happiness and renewal
- Piece of paper and a pen
- 1 small pink votive candle for emotional healing and self-esteem
- 1 teaspoon dried basil for optimism and hope
- 1 teaspoon dried rosemary for strength and healing
- 1 teaspoon dried nettle for joy and love
- 1 pink pouch for self-love

Steps to Take

1. Cleanse, ground, and center as needed.

2. Wait until sunset and choose your favorite space in your home. Prepare your materials, position yourself comfortably, and light your incense.

3. Try to relax your mind and your physical body so that you aren't holding excess tension, bringing yourself into a calm and balanced state as much as possible.

4. Take your paper and pen, draw a heart on it, and place it in the center of your workspace.

5. Now take your candle and place it directly on top of the heart.

6. Take each of the herbs and sprinkle them in a circle around your candle and recite the following as you sprinkle each:

> *Sacred basil, bring me hope for better days.*
> *Sacred rosemary, bring me strength to release my pain and begin to heal.*
> *Sacred nettle, bring me joy and love for myself.*

7. Light your candle and stare into the flame. Allow the powerful transformational energy of the fire to warm your heart and open your mind. Focus your thoughts first on the feelings of pain, doubt, and sadness—all of the emotions that are dragging you down into this place of despair. Acknowledge these feelings. Sit with them and accept them. They are a part of you and have led you to become who you are, but you must now allow them to become a part of your past. It is time to move forward. With love and kindness, allow yourself to let these feelings go and say, "With love in my heart, I accept these feelings as a part of my past and am now moving on." Find a sense of peace and empowerment when you say these words.

8. Now focus on the pink wax of your candle and allow your thoughts to shift toward everything in your life, no matter how small, that you remember bringing you joy. It can be anything at all, such as your cat, your favorite food, your witchcraft practice, or your ability to be kind even when you are feeling low. At this point the wax from your candle will be dripping. Imagine each drip of the candle is a thing in your life that has made you smile. Actively think of things and assign one to each of the candle drips. The dripping of the wax onto the heart you drew earlier represents your opening up, clearing away the darker energies within, and making space to allow these things to once again bring joy into your life. If you can, stay in this space until your candle burns down fully.

9. Once your candle is out and the wax is dried on your heart drawing,

brush the circle of herbs onto the paper and fold it up carefully with the wax and herbs inside.

10. Gently place the paper with its contents into your pink pouch and tie it up. Recite the following:

Feelings that were dark are now replaced with light.
My heart and mind are open to the future being bright.
My will inside is strong, moving on from the past.
Let my suffering be gone; this darkness shall not last.
As it is said, so mote it be.

11. Keep this pouch close and even consider carrying it with you if you are having a tough day as a reminder of your strength and the good that is in your life.

Sometimes finding clarity in the bustling space that is your mind can be challenging. There are times when making even the simplest decision may seem like an impossible task. When your mind is feeling open and clear, that will translate into other areas of your life as well. You will feel happier and more confident, and your magical work will produce strong results. But when your mind is feeling fuzzy or somehow blocked, this can lead to unnecessary stress and tension in the body. The following practices will help bring your mind to a place that is luminous and unclouded so you can clear away the fog and get your thoughts in order.

Citrus Spray to Eliminate Brain Fog

Brain fog can hit you at the most unexpected times. Maybe you didn't sleep well, have too many things going on at once, or are still recovering from a particularly draining spell. This spray will help to clear the fog from your mind and bring the world, and your tasks at hand, back into focus.

Materials to Gather

- 4-ounce dark glass spray bottle
- 1/2 teaspoon vegetable glycerin
- 15 drops lemon essential oil for awareness
- 9 drops lime essential oil for happiness
- 6 drops sweet orange essential oil for clarity
- 2 tablespoons witch hazel
- 1/3 cup distilled water

Steps to Take

1. Cleanse, ground, and center as needed.

2. Choose your workspace. Making this up in the kitchen is practical for easy cleanup and access to tools, but you may choose wherever suits you.

3. Clear your mind and prepare your ingredients. Relax your shoulders and bring attention to your center. Focus your mind on being clear and free from scattered thoughts. As you go through the steps, imagine the fog

you feel in your mind begin to lift up and away, dissipating out of the top of your head.

4. First add the vegetable glycerin into your bottle.

5. Then add in each essential oil individually and recite the following lines as you drop in each one:

> *Lemon, bring me awareness.*
> *Lime, bring me happiness.*
> *Sweet orange, bring me clarity.*

6. Now add in the witch hazel and distilled water, then place the top on.

7. Shake the bottle and recite the following:

> *Clear my mind and lift this fog.*
> *Set me free and release the smog.*
> *Clarity and focus, I can see.*
> *As my will, so mote it be.*

8. Spray three times within your space and breathe in deeply whenever you are feeling like your mind is fuzzy and not able to focus. Shake prior to each use.

Simple Decision-Making Ritual

Some days merely choosing what crystals to take with you can seem impossible. Days like this tend to happen when you are preoccupied or feeling bothered by something else that has nothing to do with the decision at hand. A little perspective and clarity are warranted in these moments, and the following spell can help get you there.

Materials to Gather

- 1 white candle for clarity
- 1 labradorite stone for awareness and intuition
- 2 pieces of paper and a pen

Steps to Take

1. Cleanse, ground, and center as needed.

2. Gather your materials and clear your mind from anything other than the decision currently at hand.

3. Place your candle in the center of your space and light it.

4. Place your labradorite stone just in front of your candle with one piece of paper on either side of it.

5. On each piece of paper write down one decision option you have been contemplating. This practice can be used for large and small decisions alike. Picture your choice in your mind's eye and think just briefly on each decision you wrote down.

6. Now place both hands above your labradorite stone and close your eyes. Say, "Labradorite, stone of the earth, bring awareness to my mind and awaken my intuition, allowing me to make the right choice for my situation."

7. With your eyes still closed, instinctively grab one of the pieces of paper. Don't allow yourself to hesitate; trust your instincts. The chosen paper will be the decision that your intuition is telling you to go with.

8. Snuff out your flame and arise from your space confident in the choice you have made.

Ritual for Clarity of Mind

Sometimes there's a lot of noise in your head and you need to clear away the cobwebs to find your way. Clarity is connected with the air element, so for this ritual you will utilize the cleansing power of air to clear away the clouds and illuminate your mind to your situation.

Materials to Gather

- Outdoor space
- 1 lapis lazuli stone for clarity and insight
- 1 labradorite stone for intuition and awareness

Steps to Take

1. Cleanse, ground, and center as needed.

2. Choose an outdoor space where you feel relaxed and comfortable. Be sure to have your two crystals with you.

3. Once you have your space, sit comfortably, hold one crystal

firmly in each hand, and take a moment to clear your mind and connect with the air element. Feel the air on your skin and the breeze rustling through the trees, and breathe deep to fill your lungs with its refreshing life-giving energy.

4. Focus your thoughts toward the situation for which you are seeking clarity.

5. Close your eyes and, either out loud or in your head, recite the following:

Lapis lazuli, bring me clarity to know what needs to be done. Labradorite, bring me awareness to trust my intuition.

Power of air, clear space in my mind to illuminate the right path.

6. Keep your eyes closed. Feel the breeze passing through you and imagine it brushing away all the fog from your mind, opening up a path of light. Visualize yourself following that path; with each step you take the path gets brighter, and when you reach the end of this path your outlook will be clear.

7. Once you finish with your visualization and you are able to see what is needed, thank the air for its service. Your work is now complete.

Memory-Boosting Tea

Peppermint is known to have positive effects on cognitive function, including memory and alertness, while lavender relaxes the nervous system. A clear and calm mind is optimal to enhance memory and learning capabilities. Magically, these herbs possess energies of happiness, renewal, cleansing, and balance—each lending itself well to forming a positive cognitive state.

Materials to Gather

- 1 cup water
- ¾ teaspoon dried peppermint for alertness and purity
- ¼ teaspoon dried lavender buds for relaxation

Steps to Take

1. Cleanse, ground, and center as needed.

2. Clear your mind and state your intention for this cup of tea

out loud, something like, "This tea will boost my memory while bringing focus and calm." Focus on holding these feelings in your mind's eye while you brew the tea.

3. Fill your pot or kettle with water and bring to a boil.

4. Add your herbs into a tea ball, teapot, or cup. As you are adding your herbs, visualize the tea doing its work. Imagine yourself retaining all the information you may be taking in with ease and confidence. You are focused and alert, and your mind is clear.

5. Once your water is boiled, pour over the herbs and let your blend steep 10–15 minutes.

6. Remove the tea ball if necessary, focus your gaze on your tea, and recite the following:

Sacred peppermint, enhance my memory and bring me focus. Sacred lavender, bring relaxation to my mind. With this spell, enhanced awareness I shall find.

7. While you drink, envision the tea expanding your mind and memory with every sip you take. Drink with intention and gratitude.

This is a great tea to have if you are studying or preparing a presentation or talk for work to help get your brain muscles in optimal shape. This blend is also delightful with a lemon wedge squeezed in once the tea is brewed.

Boosting production of dopamine and serotonin can go a long way in contributing to maintaining a positive outlook on life and encouraging a healthy state of mind. Low production of these hormones can lead to irritability, depression, difficulties learning, fatigue, and impairment of your ability to be motivated. Including boosting these happy hormones as an intention in your magical practice and making some key changes to your routine will go a long way in improving your state of mind and your ability to lead a balanced, healthy, and happy life.

Nourishing Hormone Smoothie

Serves 1

A little boost of dopamine and solid nutrition in the morning are always good ideas. Vitamin and mineral deficiencies, along with hormone imbalance, within the body can lead to poor cognitive function, anxiety, and depression. The ingredients here such as berries, coconut, and cacao are also imbued with energetic properties of joy, luck, energy, love, and abundance, all working together with vital nutrients to nourish your body and your mind.

Materials to Gather

- ½ cup coconut kefir
- ½ cup filtered water
- 1 medium banana, peeled
- ¼ cup blueberries
- ¼ cup raspberries
- 2 teaspoons all-natural almond butter
- 1 tablespoon cacao nibs
- 1 teaspoon Ceylon cinnamon
- 1 teaspoon ground flaxseed
- 1 handful spinach (or kale)
- 1 scoop high-quality protein powder (optional)

Steps to Take

1. Add all ingredients into a blender in the order listed. As you are adding each ingredient, concentrate on the fresh whole ingredients and the positive effects they will have on your body. They are providing you vital

nutrients that will help to boost your overall mood and nourish your cells. Envision yourself going through your day happy, positive, and smiling and feeling light on your feet.

2. Hold this vision of your joy-filled day in your mind and blend the ingredients for 30–60 seconds.

3. Once the ingredients are blended, pour the mixture into your glass and recite the following:

Happiness and positivity, come my way.
Smiles and joy, please fill my day.
Nourishing and healthy whole food,
benefit my mind and boost my mood.

4. Don't forget to give thanks to the earth for this uplifting beverage and enjoy!

Enchanting a Pendant for Joy and Luck

Wearing your magic in the form of beautiful jewelry isn't a new concept. For centuries jewelry has been worn for magical and mystical purposes. In this ritual, you will embrace this ancient practice and craft a pendant for joy and luck. The knowledge that you're wearing something imbued with magical intentions will serve to bring further feelings of happiness and confidence to you. Begin this ritual on a Thursday, an optimal day for magic related to joy and happiness.

Materials to Gather

- Bowl of water
- 1 pink candle for happiness
- 1 orange candle for luck
- Clean cloth
- Pin or ritual knife
- 1 moonstone, amethyst stone, or carnelian stone with a bale so that it may fit on a necklace
- 1 chain, ribbon, or cord to place the stone on

Steps to Take

1. Cleanse, ground, and center as needed.

2. Choose your workspace. If you don't have an altar, choose a space where you are able to leave your candles and bowl of water for the full week. Clear your mind. Bring your mind into a space of light, joy, and positivity. Try not to allow any negative thoughts in.

3. Set up your supplies with your bowl of water in the center of your space, flanked by your candles on either side. Lay your clean cloth out flat in front of your bowl and place your stone and necklace on top of it.

4. On the pink candle, carve in the word "joy" with your pin or knife and then light the candle. On the orange candle, carve the word "luck" and then light it.

5. Slide your stone onto your chosen necklace material. Hold it out in front of you and say, "This pendant will bring to me joy and luck."

6. Now gently dip the necklace into the water and place it back in front of the bowl.

7. Close your eyes, place both hands above the necklace, and recite the following:

> *Joy and luck will come my way.*
> *Be it night or be it day.*
> *From the sky above to the earth below.*
> *Pendant, allow these energies to flow.*

8. Open your eyes and thank the elements for their aid, then fold the sides of your cloth over the pendant.

9. Each day extinguish your candles and leave everything set just as it is and each day at the same time relight your candles and repeat steps 5–7 for the next 6 days. Then on the following day, which will again be the Thursday, you can begin to wear your newly charmed pendant.

Spell Jar for Happiness

Spell jars are extremely versatile and can be used for almost any intention simply by changing up the ingredients. With this practice you'll craft a happiness jar. Placing this jar in a prominent space where you sometimes may need a little pick-me-up is good practice, and always feel free to make more than one if needed.

Materials to Gather

- Yellow candle to encourage optimism
- 1 tablespoon dried chamomile to uplift the mood
- 1 tablespoon dried catnip for happiness and beauty
- 1 tablespoon dried basil for hope
- Small glass Mason jar with lid
- 1 carnelian stone for positivity
- 3 drops lemon essential oil for joy
- 1 yellow string or ribbon, long enough to tie around jar

Steps to Take

1. Cleanse, ground, and center as needed.

2. Choose your workspace and gather your materials. Allow your mind to be at ease. Begin to think happy thoughts. What things in your life bring you happiness? What are you looking forward to in the days to come? Shift your thoughts to this lighter frame of mind.

3. Sit comfortably to promote relaxation and light your candle.

4. Clear your head and focus your mind on feelings of joy, happiness, optimism, hope, and the beauty that is this life you were given—feelings that are extremely easy to lose sight of.

5. Add in each herb individually into your jar. Visualize the energy of indisputable joy surrounding your entire body in a beautiful yellow hue, infusing you with positivity and uplifting energies. You have many things in your life that bring you happiness. Let these things fill your mind.

6. Add in your carnelian stone and essential oil. Recite the following:

*Feelings of optimism within shall
reign.
Peace and light flow through
my veins.
Joy inside a powerful shift.
Each new day a raw sweet gift.
As my will, so mote it be.*

7. Close up your jar and tie your yellow string in a bow around the top of the jar.

8. Place your jar in front of your candle and focus on the flame through the glass. Keep your visualization strong in your mind. Say, "I choose to be happy and positive." You may now extinguish your flame.

9. Place the jar in a place of prominence where you will regularly see it.

Tea Ritual to Promote Happiness

Happy teas are a wonderful addition to any witch's cupboard, and it's great to have a few recipes on hand to use when you're feeling down or just a little blue. This tea is perfect for moments when this type of mood strikes.

Materials to Gather

- 1 cup water
- ¾ teaspoon dried lemongrass
- ¼ teaspoon dried sage

Steps to Take

1. Clear your mind and state your intention for this cup of tea out loud, something like, "This tea will boost my mood and bring me joy." Focus on holding these feelings in your heart while you brew the tea.

2. Fill your pot or kettle with water and bring to a boil.

3. Add your herbs into a tea ball, teapot, or mug. As you are adding your herbs, visualize the tea literally transforming into joyful energy. Continue to hold feelings of happiness and positivity in your mind, allow yourself to feel relaxed, and let a smile come to your lips.

4. Once your water is boiled, pour it over the herbs and let your blend steep for 10–15 minutes.

5. Remove the tea ball if necessary, focus your gaze on your tea, and recite the following:

Sacred lemongrass, cleanse my mind and boost my mood.

Sacred sage, bring joy and lift my spirits well.
I give thanks for your aid, to bring happiness with this spell.

6. While you drink, envision the tea boosting your outlook as you sip. Drink with intention and gratitude.

This is a great tea to have first thing in the morning as a nice boost to your day. This blend is also delightful with a lemon wedge squeezed in once the tea is brewed.

For many witches, their coven is their family, those they turn to for strength, support, and love. This type of bond creates powerful magic within your community and in your own individual practice. Fostering these healthy and positive relationships in your life is integral to your overall sense of well-being. Everyone needs people in their life to talk to, connect with, and bond with. Surrounding yourself with a community of individuals that you communicate well with and who share your interests can lower your stress and contribute to positive emotions such as joy, confidence, and positivity. A lack of these connections in your life can lead to low moods, higher levels of stress, and an impaired immune system.

Utilizing your craft to encourage positive relationships in your life and to let go of those that inflict negativity is most worthy magical work. When performing this type of magic, you are not in any way affecting the other person's free will or state of mind. The following rituals are focused only on you and your own personal growth.

Ritual to Release Toxic Relationships

While a positive relationship can lift you up, a toxic one can tear you down and make you feel small, insecure, and unworthy of something better. Coming to terms with these toxic relationships will enable you to accept things for what they were and move on to more fulfilling engagements. Use this ritual to let go and free yourself from any chains still in place.

Materials to Gather

- 1 stick eucalyptus incense for banishing and cleansing
- 2 black tourmaline stones for strength and healing
- 4 pieces of black string or thread (1 longer than the others)
- Scissors
- Cauldron, firesafe dish, or trowel

Steps to Take

1. Cleanse, ground, and center as needed.

2. Choose your workspace and gather your materials.

3. Place your incense in the center of your space, then place one black tourmaline stone on either side. Lay out the four strings in front of your incense burner, with the long one at the back. Now light your incense.

4. Close your eyes and think about the relationship you are letting go of. Consider and reaffirm with yourself all the reasons why the relationship has come to an end and how the relationship made you feel. What emotions are you still hanging on to? Are you feeling anger, betrayal, hurt, sadness? Choose the three emotions that you are suffering from the most.

5. Now pick up your first string and say, for example, "I release anger." Replace "anger" with whatever emotion you are letting go of by releasing this relationship. Now cut the thread in half and place each piece on opposite sides of your workspace. Repeat this for the next two threads.

6. Now take the longer thread, hold it out in front of you, and say "I release this relationship and am ready to move on." Now cut the thread in half and add the pieces with the others.

7. To dispose of the threads, you can either burn them in your cauldron or firesafe dish and dispose of the ashes or take the two piles of threads and bury them in opposite ends of your yard to signify that they will never be fused back together. Allow your incense to burn down fully.

Ritual to Foster Healthy Relationships

You undoubtedly want to have strong and positive relationships in your life that fuel you and make you feel like a better version of yourself. However, it's not always easy to connect or find people you feel an affinity with. This ritual works to draw these types of relationships into your life and to strengthen ones that are already there.

Materials to Gather

- 1 pink candle for friendship and love
- Mortar and pestle
- ½ cup sugar for love and sweetness
- 1 tablespoon dried hibiscus for passion
- 1 tablespoon dried nettle for happiness
- 1 tablespoon dried valerian for harmony
- Medium Mason jar with lid
- 1 each of rose quartz, amethyst, and rhodochrosite stones to encourage healthy, positive relationships
- 1 pink ribbon

Steps to Take

1. Cleanse, ground, and center as needed.

2. Sit comfortably in your space, relax your mind, and light your candle.

3. Take your mortar and add in the sugar and then each one of the herbs and begin to blend all together with your pestle. As you blend, visualize the relationships in your life growing, prospering, and thriving, or imagine beautiful new relationships that are healthy and positive entering your life. Visualize what will work best for your situation right now; you could focus on one particular relationship or many. Continue with this as you blend for a couple of minutes. Hold on to the feelings the images invoke in you and keep the images in your mind.

4. Add the mixture into your jar and one by one add in your three crystals. Tie your pink ribbon into a circle to represent unity and place it into the jar last.

5. Place your hands over the top of the jar and recite the following:

I open my life to those who deserve me.
Creating joyful and light energy.
Loving, happy, and positive bonds.
Goddess, bring me relationships that are healthy and strong.

6. Place the lid on your jar and extinguish your flame. Set the jar on your altar or other place of prominence.

Journaling Ritual for Self-Discovery

Your most important relationship in life is the one you have with yourself. Cultivating this is integral before you're able to encourage strong and thriving relationships with others. The following ritual will encourage you to dig deep, get to know yourself better, and bring all the things that make you so brilliant into the light.

Materials to Gather

- A notebook that you love
- A special pen

Steps to Take

1. Cleanse, ground, and center as needed.

2. Gather your supplies and relax into your space. Give yourself at least 30 minutes to complete this ritual. You don't want to rush the process.

3. Clear your mind and focus on you. You are the sole subject of this exercise. Here you will write an ode and a spell to yourself.

4. Begin to write down all the qualities that you possess within yourself, both positive and less so, as well as things you enjoy and excel at or have tried and failed at. This exercise is about knowing and getting comfortable with yourself. We are all human with human talents, flaws, and personalities. Now think back to when you were a child. What positive and not so positive attributes did you have then? What were your favorite things?

What things were you excited to try? Then move on and repeat the same for your teen, young adult, and adult years. You are writing down an evolution of yourself. How have you changed and who is the person that stares back at you from the mirror today? Really dig deep and let everything you can think of come out onto the paper.

The final section in your writing will describe the empowered, strong, and magical human being you have grown into today.

5. This is a great piece of writing that you can refer back to when you may feel a little lost and need a reminder of the unique and special individual you are now and always have been.

Candle Ritual for Encouraging Love

There is always room for more love in life. Pink, vanilla, and the powerful warmth of fire all come together in this candle ritual to harness loving energies and to encourage more of it to enter your life. Friday, the day of Venus, is an optimal day to perform love magic.

Materials to Gather

- 1 pink candle for love and friendship
- 1 stick vanilla incense for love and beauty

Steps to Take

1. Cleanse, ground, and center as needed.

2. Choose a quiet place in your home where you will not be disturbed. Center yourself and clear your mind.

3. Sit comfortably, then light your candle and incense.

4. Take three deep breaths and focus your gaze on the flame. Visualize a vibrant pink ray of light rising up from the flame and

creating a beautifully bright pink aura around yourself.

5. Close your eyes and recite the following:

> Sacred flame, bring love to me.
> I open my heart; I release the key.
> I open my eyes and relax my mind.
> Inside, it's love that I shall find.

6. Open your eyes, give thanks to the fire element, and say, "So mote it be."

7. You may now extinguish your flame. Keep this image of the bright pink aura around yourself and come back to it when you are meeting new people or spending time with friends.

The following rituals are here to help you further explore different areas of your mental and emotional wellness. From creativity to protection for empaths, they will assist in opening your mind and easing emotional tensions.

Ring Ritual for Enhancing Creativity

Everyone should have something in their life that lets their creative side shine. Your creativity may sometimes need help to flow freely. This ring can be worn to help you tap in to those energies when they are lacking and need a little help getting out.

Materials to Gather

- 1 orange candle for creativity
- Tongs
- 1 silver ring
- 1 drop jasmine essential oil (properly diluted) for creativity and confidence

Steps to Take

1. Cleanse, ground, and center as needed.

2. Choose a space in your home where you feel joyful and free. Take a breath and relax your energies. For creativity to flow effortlessly, your mind must be clear and free from stresses. Let everything go and focus on the ritual at hand.

3. Light your candle and say, "Blessed flame, transform this ring into a beacon of creativity and light."

4. Use the tongs to pick up the ring and pass it through the flame one time, then set the ring down in front of the candle.

5. Place a drop of the jasmine essential oil on your index finger and anoint the ring with it, being careful to check that the ring is sufficiently cooled down. Say, "Sacred jasmine, gift of the earth, bring confidence to my creative self."

6. Now place the ring on your finger, close your palm, and let

your other hand lay on top of the ring. Recite the following:

Creativity, come to me.
Open my mind and set it free.
Earth and fire, hear my call.
May my muse never fall.
And so, it is done.

7. You may now extinguish your flame. Wear this ring whenever you are working on a project that requires your creative energies to be flowing freely; this may be every day or just once in a while. Keep the ring in a safe, protected space when you're not wearing it.

Reveal Unseen Truths Through Water Scrying

If you feel like something is being kept from you, it can be draining mentally and emotionally. In this practice, you may focus on any situation in your life where a lack of transparency may be plaguing you. Scrying can be a difficult medium, so don't be discouraged if you need to repeat this a few times. When scrying, you're possibly making yourself vulnerable to outside spiritual influences, making it wise to ground yourself prior to beginning and to have something in your space for protection, such as casting a circle or using a protective crystal as we do here. Perform this during a full moon, a powerful time for divination practices. Otherwise, a Wednesday also works well as it carries strong magical influence for divination work of any kind.

Materials to Gather

- 1 clean blue cloth for intuition and spiritual awareness
- 1 bowl of water
- 3 lapis lazuli stones for truth and insight
- 1 black tourmaline stone for protection
- 1 stick frankincense incense to reveal truths
- Notebook and a pen

Steps to Take

1. Choose a quiet space where you will not be disturbed and clear your mind. You want your mind to be open and free from distractions so that you are open to receive messages and the truth that may come to you.

2. Place the blue cloth in the center of your space and set the bowl of water on top of it, then

gently place your four stones around your bowl, with the black tourmaline in the bottom position closest to you.

3. Light your incense and circle it around clockwise and over the cloth and dish of water, then place it behind your dish of water.

4. Recite your intention, something like, "I open my mind to truths unseen."

5. Focus your mind and ensure it is clear of any outside thoughts or distractions. Relax the muscles in your body and concentrate on deep, steady breathing. Set your gaze on the water and work to relax into your own intuition and spiritual awareness. What images or visions are you seeing in the water's surface? What thoughts are forming in your mind? These are messages trying to get through; be open to them and trust your instincts in the process. Take your time with this step as it may take several minutes for anything to begin to take shape. Stay in this space until you feel satisfied with your outcome.

6. You may wish to record in your journal anything that you see or think during your session so you don't forget important details. Have patience and you may realize the truth was inside you all along and this was just what was needed to bring it to the surface. Allow your incense to burn down fully if safe to do so.

Protection Ritual for Empaths

Being an empath can be a wonderful but tiring gift. While it's remarkable to be able to read people and tap in to their emotions, it can also be emotionally draining. For many empaths, simply being in a crowded environment can be overwhelming and exhausting. Creating a protection barrier can help to ease the strain and protect your mind.

Materials to Gather

- 1 black candle for protection
- 1 black pouch for protection and release
- 1 tablespoon dried rosemary for protection and strength
- 3 amethyst stones for protection and positivity
- 3 drops patchouli essential oil for protection and grounding

Steps to Take

1. Cleanse, ground, and center as needed.

2. Find a space where you feel relaxed and will not be disturbed. Sit comfortably and light your candle.

3. Clear your mind, breathe deep, slow your heart rate, relax your shoulders, and try to feel a sense of calm washing over you. Your mind should be free from excess stress while completing this ritual as you are working here to protect your sensitive emotions.

4. Take your pouch, add in the rosemary, and say, "Rosemary of the earth, give me strength to protect my mind."

5. Add in your amethyst stones one at a time and say, "Amethyst stones, power of the earth, bring me positive energy to combat negative surroundings."

6. Add in the essential oil and say, "Sacred patchouli, ground my energy so that I may remain balanced and calm."

7. Now tie up your pouch, hold it to your heart, and say:

> Earth energies, bring protection to my mind,
> block the emotions I do not wish to find.
> Grounded and calm for all to see,
> as my will, so mote it be.

8. It is best to carry this pouch with you, especially when you will be in situations where you know there will be a lot of negativity or overwhelming energies such as crowded spaces or places with somber energy.

Ritual to Boost Motivation

Motivation can sometimes be elusive. You awaken feeling good and determined to have a productive day, and then as the day goes on, the motivation slowly dissipates until it's difficult to get anything done. This ritual will give your motivation a boost.

Materials to Gather

- 1 stick bergamot incense for confidence and motivation
- Small decorative box
- Items that represent your specific goals
- 1 each of carnelian, tiger's eye, and red jasper stones for motivation

Steps to Take

1. Cleanse, ground, and center as needed.

2. Relax into your space and center your mind. Light your incense and focus on your feelings of determination, motivation, and vibrant energy.

3. Take your box and begin adding in your personal items relating to your goals. As you do this, visualize yourself working hard to make these goals a reality. Imagine what your life will look like once you are able to fully manifest these dreams. How will you feel and how will your life change?

4. After those items are all added, place your three crystals on top and close the box.

5. Take your incense stick and trace the outside of the box, letting the smoke wash over the sides and top. As you do this, recite the following:

> *Motivation strong and sound.*
> *Focus within from sky to ground.*
> *My mind determined three times three.*
> *As my will, so mote it be.*

6. Place the box on your dresser or altar, and each morning, place your hands atop the box and say, "I am motivated and determined to reach my goals." Allow your incense to burn down fully if safe to do so.

7. You may repeat this ritual to update your box whenever your goals change and evolve.

MENTAL WELLNESS JOURNAL PROMPTS AND AFFIRMATIONS

These prompts and affirmations will help to bring clarity to your thoughts and feelings, help you to stay on track with your goals when it comes to fostering a healthy mindset, and encourage you to use writing as a therapeutic tool.

Journal Prompts for Mental and Emotional Wellness

1. Write down five of your favorite inspirational quotes and why they speak to you.

2. What are the top three things in your life that bring you happiness? Write about each one and what about them makes you so happy.

3. What is your biggest fear that you wish you could overcome and what is the first thing you would want to do if you could?

4. Write a letter to yourself. In the letter let yourself know what you love about yourself, things you forgive yourself for, and anything else you want yourself to know.

5. Think about someone from your past that has caused you emotional trauma. If you could have a conversation with them tomorrow, what are some things you would like to say?

Daily Affirmations for Mental and Emotional Wellness

- I am a strong and powerful witch.

- I am motivated and inspired.

- My mind is free from emotional traumas.

- I release negative thought patterns.

- I embrace positivity and happiness.

Your journey toward wellness is an ever changing one. We are all on different paths and have our own versions of what being well looks like. No matter what point you may be at in your own journey your magic is worthy and valid. No ailment, be it mental or physical, can take away from that. You are your own brand of magic and that is something to be cherished.

CHAPTER FIVE

Magic for Spiritual Wellness

Your spirit is your life force, energy, drive, and ultimate inner power. To nurture your spirit is to bring clarity, mindfulness, and purpose to your greater self, and to be more fully in touch with your true self. Practicing spiritual wellness is tending to your innermost desires, following your dreams, finding true peace, and having a clear vision of who you are and what you need to feel whole.

Your witchcraft practice is an integral part of your spirituality. Tending to and connecting with your spirit can provide a sense of comfort, connect you with your purpose, and help you to better understand your experiences. This chapter will explore some different ways to connect to your spiritual wellness, such as balancing energies, connecting to nature, opening yourself up to new possibilities, trusting your intuition, and working with the elements and universe in your practice.

Your spirit is the very essence of who you are; it is your inner soul and magic. Taking charge and nurturing this very core piece of yourself will have benefits that spill over into all parts of your life. You will feel more in sync with your own wants and needs, be more aligned with your environment and surroundings, and be an overall stronger witch, both in your health and magic. When you are truly in touch with your spirit and your most inner self, that is when your magic and your spell work can flourish, bringing your witchcraft abilities to new heights.

The beautiful journey of transformation for your spirit may possibly be the most rewarding on your magical wellness journey. The following spells and rituals are essentials as you journey inward to awaken your spirit.

Spell Collage to Connect with Your Authentic Self

Everyone is always telling you to be yourself, but we are often out of touch with who we truly are. Your authentic self has nothing to do with your job or other people in your life, but the essence that is you, at your deepest, most vulnerable, and most powerful: the way you think, the things you like, and the way you act, without any filters to please others.

Getting in touch with your authentic self can help to feed your spirit and awaken or reawaken parts of yourself that have been pushed beneath the surface. It can help you realize your passions and dreams, and discover which road is right for you to travel down at this moment. Creating this collage will help you reflect on who your authentic self truly is.

Materials to Gather

- 1 purple candle for wisdom and connection to your higher self
- 1 stick eucalyptus incense for growth
- 3 labradorite stones for self-discovery, creativity, and awareness
- Piece of paper, at least 8" × 10" in size
- Pen
- Magazines, pictures, newspapers, and so on
- Scissors
- Glue or tape

Steps to Take

1. Cleanse, ground, and center as needed.

2. Prepare your supplies and choose a space where you will feel comfortable and relaxed.

3. Calm your mind and clear it of any distractions. This is not the time to think about to-do lists, or work, or bills. These next few minutes are about only you, a time to focus on the things you like and dislike and your own opinions and thoughts. This collage is for you and you alone.

4. Light your candle and incense, then place your labradorite stones evenly around your workspace.

5. Take your pen and write the following words in the center of your paper:

My inner self be sight and seen.
From here to there, and in between.
My inner self, shine bright and true.
Authentically me through and through.

6. This is your spell and mantra to yourself to not hide who you are but to let your authenticity shine bright in everything you do. This is a commitment to yourself to learn who you truly are and to not dampen your spirit for anyone or anything. Embrace becoming the witch you were always meant to be.

7. Now begin to go through the magazines and pictures you've gathered. There is no plan here; you simply need to cut out any images or words that speak to you. Look for things that make you smile or have you feeling passionate, such as an outfit, a powerful phrase, a piece of art—anything at all. Once you find an image that calls to you, cut it out and paste it on the page in whatever manner feels correct. There is no pattern to collage; simply place the images in a way that feels right. Continue cutting and pasting your images until you have filled your page. Every image on it should speak to your inner self. You should be able to say, "Yes, I love this" or "Yes, this is important to me." The end collage should be a true representation of you.

8. You may extinguish your incense and candle; there is no need to let them burn down unless you would like to. You may bring them out to use again if you repeat this exercise or for similar magical

work. Place the collage on your refrigerator or in an area where you will see it often as a reminder to yourself that you know who you are and you are not afraid to always be that person.

9. We are always learning new things about ourselves. It may be good practice to repeat this collage activity once a month to continue learning and discovering new things about yourself. You may surprise yourself and be pulled to include images you didn't necessarily think represented you in the past. Things that speak to you will evolve over time, and it's nice to be in touch enough with yourself to recognize these changes. These collages can help make apparent to you the things that truly speak to your heart.

Meditation to Find Your True Purpose

There may be times you feel lost, directionless, or confused, as though you're simply going through the motions of life with no real passion or purpose. Having a strong sense of purpose in life will help ward off illness, give you a powerful sense of direction in your witchcraft practice, and provide you with a strong sense of self and identity.

Materials to Gather

- 1 stick peppermint incense for renewal
- 2 clear quartz stones for awareness and clarity

Steps to Take

1. Cleanse, ground, and center as needed.

2. Choose a quiet space where you will not be disturbed. Relax your mind and light your incense.

3. Sit comfortably, take your two crystals and hold one in each hand, and close your eyes. Take a few concentrated breaths. Focus on making them slow, deep,

and steady. Now think for a few minutes on the different aspects of your life. What are your job and homelife like? Do you have any hobbies? Try and think of which aspects of your life bring you happiness and make you smile and which things you could really do without. What are the things that you do because you genuinely want to and what things do you do out of obligation?

4. Hone in on the things that make you feel happiest, most alive, and full of energy. These are the things that give you life and feed your soul, and these are the things that your life should be dominated by. Focus on these aspects and visualize what your life would be like if you could release the things in your life you are not passionate about or do solely out of obligation.

What would it take to redesign your life to have it centered around the things that make you feel complete?

5. Stay in your meditation, holding this visualization and imagining how different things could be. What pieces of the visualization are dominating your thoughts and tugging at your emotions? Tapping in to and acknowledging these things will start you on a path to living life with purpose, passion, and vitality.

6. Stay in your meditative state for 10–15 minutes. Allow your incense to burn down fully if possible. Once you finish, you may find it beneficial to record your thoughts and feelings around it in your journal or grimoire. Repeating this meditation once a week will help you to create a clearer picture of what best to focus on in your life.

Ritual for Appreciating Your Spirit Self

You may often show gratitude for the many gifts in your life, but do you ever take the time to appreciate your spiritual self, the part of yourself that connects you with the universe, your intuition, and your inner wisdom? It's easy to forget to show appreciation for, and truly see, this aspect of yourself. The following ritual will assist in showing some love to this important side of you.

Materials to Gather

- 1 purple candle for spirituality and connection to your higher self
- 2 lapis lazuli stones for wisdom and insight

Steps to Take

1. Cleanse, ground, and center as needed.

2. Choose a location you feel relaxed and sit comfortably. Now arrange your materials with the candle in the middle and the stones flanking it on either side. Take a deep breath and clear your mind.

3. Light your candle and focus your gaze on the flame and hold one palm above each of your stones to help absorb their energies into yourself.

4. Your spirit is the very essence of you, so think to yourself what color would you be if you were a color. Now visualize yourself being surrounded by and enveloped in a brilliant hue of this particular color.

Imagine the color surrounding not only your physical body but also permeating within you because your spirit exists in every part of yourself. Allow yourself to feel love, appreciation, and gratitude for this beautiful light that is you. Your spirit is vibrant, strong, and unique. Think of words you would use to describe your spirit and take a moment to appreciate them.

5. Your energy should be feeling empowered and humbled in this moment. Recite the following:

You are my light; you are my heart.
Always unique, and never apart.
My true essence, deep within.
There for me, you've always been.

6. You may now lower your hands. Give one final thanks to your spirit for guiding you through this magical journey of life. You may now extinguish your flame.

Spell Jar to Access Your Inner Wisdom

We all have untapped wisdom inside of us, knowledge of ourselves, our intuition, and truths we may not want to see. If you look inside yourself and allow access to these hidden pieces of information, you will grow and flourish into the healthiest, most powerful witch you can possibly be. This spell jar will serve to help connect with these inner elements of yourself.

Materials to Gather

- Small Mason jar with lid
- 1 purple candle for wisdom and purpose
- 1 blue candle for insight and intuition
- 3 tablespoons dried sage for wisdom, cleansing, and mental clarity
- 1 amethyst stone for wisdom
- 1 black tourmaline stone for grounding
- 1 lapis lazuli stone for truth
- 3 drops sandalwood essential oil for peace and clarity
- 1 purple ribbon to represent your higher self

Steps to Take

1. Cleanse, ground, and center as needed.

2. Clear your mind, sit comfortably in your space, and direct your thoughts inward.

3. Set your Mason jar in the middle of your space with one candle on either side.

4. Light your candles. Focus on freeing and opening up your mind to your innermost thoughts. Allow yourself to think about things you generally wouldn't think about or a specific topic on your mind that you require some direction with. Keep your mind calm and at peace with whatever thoughts begin to flow. Stay away from focusing on the everyday things like to-do lists and appointments.

5. Put the dried sage into the jar, then your crystals and essential oil. While filling your jar, focus on keeping your mind open and connected to your deepest thoughts and knowledge.

6. Lastly, tie the ends of your ribbon together so that it forms a circle. This represents the

continuous circle of your higher self, always within you waiting to be accessed. Place the ribbon inside the jar and close the lid.

7. Place both hands above the jar, close your eyes, and recite the following three times:

I will look within; let my inner wisdom speak and I will listen.

8. You may now extinguish your flames and place the jar in your bedroom so that you may see it each morning when you rise and every evening when you go to bed as a reminder that wisdom and knowledge reside inside of you, always.

Meditation for Inner Peace

Attaining inner peace allows you to maintain a sense of calm and balance regardless of what may be happening in your life. Finding true inner peace will lower anxiety and stress in the body and allow you to react to different situations with ease and clarity. The more you practice, the more often your body will naturally shift into this state.

Materials to Gather

- 1 stick lavender incense for peace and calm

Steps to Take

1. Cleanse, ground, and center as needed.

2. Choose a quiet space where you will not be disturbed, relax your mind, and light your incense.

3. Sit comfortably and close your eyes. Take a few moments to concentrate on regulating your breathing to attain a smooth and steady state. Take long, deep inhales and relaxed exhales. Now focus on letting go of any emotions or thoughts that are bringing you out of a calm place. Release them out into the air. Those thoughts do not serve you in this space.

4. Now in the center of your forehead imagine a soft, glowing blue light forming. Visualize this light moving inward through your forehead and flowing smoothly

down throughout your entire body. Allow the vision of the blue light to extend beyond your physical self and to surround you with a blue peaceful aura. Once you can fully envision yourself enveloped by this blue essence, recite the following in your mind:

Spirit calm and harmony within. Balance and peace surround my skin.

5. Stay in your meditation, holding this luminous image in your mind, and repeat the deep breathing for a few moments as you did in the beginning. Once finished, open your eyes, snuff out your candle, and say, "So mote it be."

Full Moon Bath to Embrace the Divine Feminine Within

The divine feminine exists within each of us regardless of gender identification and is a powerful part of any witchcraft practice. Feminine energy is strongly connected to the moon and Mother Earth. Connecting with this energy can help characteristics of yourself emerge that may have become buried over time. This can increase joy, enhance intuition, ease anxiety, and open yourself to love and compassion. This ritual will focus on self-love, allowing you to gain insight into your divine feminine side.

Materials to Gather

- 2 silver candles to represent the moon and intuition
- 1 stick vanilla incense for gentle feminine energy
- ½ cup Himalayan pink salt for love
- 6 drops geranium essential oil for honesty
- 3 drops rose essential oil for compassion

Steps to Take

1. Cleanse, ground, and center as needed.

2. Relax your mind while preparing for your ritual. Take your time to set up your materials, lay out something made of soft, luxurious material to put on afterward, and add in any special touches you wish to include to help set the mood, such as soothing music, a favorite beverage, or flowers.

3. Once your space is prepared, light your candles and incense and begin to run your bath.

4. While the water is running, slowly add in your ingredients one at a time in the order they are listed. During this process, bring your energy to a place that feels calm, accepting, loving, and open. These are traits that are inherently feminine. Bringing yourself into this space will help to connect your spirit to the feminine energy within.

5. When the bathtub is sufficiently filled, turn the water off, gently step into the tub, and settle yourself comfortably. Take a few moments here to close your eyes and think of your own qualities that are feminine in nature; remember, we all have feminine qualities regardless of gender identity. Are you nurturing, creative, empathetic, sensitive, or understanding? Compile a list of qualities in your mind.

6. Commit to acknowledging and nurturing these qualities as you move forward. Allow yourself to embrace and feel these characteristics as part of your divine spirit. Recite the following:

> *Feminine beauty, open and strong.*
> *I feel, I hear, the moon's gentle song.*
> *This power inside, I now fully see.*
> *This is my word, so mote it be.*

7. Spend as much time as you like relaxing in this space and frame of mind. Once you feel complete, extinguish your candles and incense, then dress and finish your day in a calm and centred manner. Simply stare at the moon, sit outside, or listen to some tranquil music, and just take in the beauty that surrounds you.

Presenting an Offering to a Deity

It's the personal choice of every witch whether or not to work with a deity. You may find working with a deity will strengthen your connection with nature and the universe and feed your spirit. Usually a connection is made organically; either you feel drawn to a deity or they call out to you, creating a more authentic relationship. Once a relationship is forged, presenting your deity with offerings is a wonderful way to solidify this bond and show your appreciation for their guidance.

Materials to Gather

- 1 white candle (or other color associated with your deity)
- Representation of your deity (this can be a statue, object, picture, etc.)
- A bowl or plate
- Small amount of bread or grains

Steps to Take

1. Cleanse, ground, and center as needed.

2. Choose a space that you can set up as an area dedicated to your deity. This can be on your altar if you have one or any small area in your home or yard that can be left set up undisturbed. You do not need much space for this.

3. Once you have chosen your space, arrange your candle and deity representation in a manner that pleases you and fits the space. Now light your candle.

4. Place the bowl in the center of the space and add in your grains.

5. Sit quietly in contemplation for a moment and close your eyes. Let your heart fill with gratitude for the divine connection you have established. Let feelings of love, thanks, and appreciation wash over you. Then state the following, "Blessed (you may insert their name here), thank you for your love and guidance as I journey down my path. I honor you and am grateful for your aid and support." You may now extinguish your flame.

6. While you need to set your space up only one time, you may give

offerings as often as you feel is right to do so. It could be once a week, every month, or on the Sabbats or any days that are associated with your deity of choice. Your relationship is yours alone, so do what feels right. Each time you complete a new offering, light your candle and give a word of thanks and gratitude to your deity. You may compost (if applicable) your previous offering when necessary.

Journaling to Access Your Shadow Self

Your shadow self is made up of the darkest parts of you that you may try to ignore or push aside. We all have light and dark within us; we all have feelings, impulses, and personality traits we'd rather we didn't. You may feel pretending these parts of yourself don't exist will make them disappear, but on the contrary, it may in fact make them more intense.

These dark parts are still aspects of what make you who you are and need to be accepted in order to truly heal. Ignoring these darker parts of yourself can lead to mental health issues, low self-esteem, insomnia, and erratic spell work. This ritual will help you to connect with and embrace your shadow self, which can also uncover hidden gifts and positive traits within.

Materials to Gather

- 1 stick peppermint incense for healing and renewal
- A journal or some blank paper
- Pen

Steps to Take

1. Choose a space that you can return to at the end of each day for the next 8 days. You will repeat this exercise at the same time for 7 days, returning on the eighth day to bring everything together. Assure you are in a good mental space when you begin. Connecting to your shadow self can be challenging and you wouldn't want the experience to have a negative effect on yourself.

2. Take a deep breath, relax your mind, and light your incense. Go over your day in your head. What reactions, emotions, and thoughts

did you have while going about your tasks and interacting with others? While you contemplate this, focus on the negative thoughts, reactions, and emotions you had.

3. Take your paper and pen and begin to record these aspects of your day from when you woke until this moment while you are writing everything out. Don't hold anything back. If you felt angry, jealous, overcritical of others, moody, arrogant, paranoid, or other similar emotions, write it down; record it all with an open and honest mind. It is okay and perfectly human to encounter these types of emotions and reactions.

4. Once you are finished writing, say, "These shadows are pieces of me. I acknowledge them as part of who I am. I am strong enough to accept them and not let them control me."

5. Repeat this exact exercise for 7 full days. You may relight your incense each day and replace as needed. On the eighth day, read back through your past 7 days of writing. Pay attention to the patterns and behaviors that tend to repeat themselves. Now take your paper and pen once again

and make a list of everything that stands out to you. Your shadow self has dominant traits and patterns. By writing these down you are allowing them to be brought into the light and enabling yourself to let go of any shame you may have attached to them.

6. Lastly, take a moment to read this new list, out loud if you are able to, and think about each thing you've written. Reflect on other times in your life these things have manifested. Maintain honesty with yourself as you go through your list. Allow the incense to burn down fully, then close your eyes and recite the following:

Shadows within flow gentle, flow free.
Calm yet chaotic, like wind and sea.
Accept and guide these parts of me.
Strong is my will, so mote it be.

7. Working with your shadow self can be a long and arduous journey. This exercise is but a starting point to begin shedding light on the traits you once wished would remain hidden from yourself but are now ready to accept. Repeat this exercise as often as needed or reread your list from day 8 and reflect.

Ritual for Releasing Guilt and Gaining Forgiveness

Forgiving yourself for behaviors, feelings, or past transgressions will enable burdens to lift. Guilt and shame weigh heavy on the spirit, and showing yourself compassion will bring you closer to accepting your own self-worth. The following ritual will enable you to release any ill-gotten feelings dampening your spirit, enabling you to move forward and grow.

Materials to Gather

- 1 black candle for banishing
- 1 red candle for courage and strength
- Piece of paper and a pen
- Cauldron or firesafe dish

Steps to Take

1. Cleanse, ground, and center as needed.

2. Clear your mind and sit relaxed in your space.

3. Set your candles side by side and light them. Focus on any actions, emotions, or thoughts that have feelings of guilt, regret, or shame attached. Allow these emotions to rise to the surface, as they have likely been pushed down and buried. Think of the instances that caused these feelings to form inside yourself. Allow yourself to be vulnerable and fully remember them. You're allowed to make mistakes; it is part of what makes you human. Accept that these things are part of your past and that you deserve the gift of forgiveness.

4. Take your paper and pen and make a list of everything you can think of for which you are offering yourself this compassion.

5. Now take the paper, use your candles to carefully light two corners, one with each flame, of the paper on fire, and drop the paper into your cauldron or firesafe dish.

6. Stare into the flame and feel your compassion and courage move forward inside yourself. As you accept forgiveness, feel the love for yourself growing and the weight of these burdens being lifted from your shoulders. Recite the following:

I've had guilt, I've had shame.
Nobody left to blame.
I love myself, I set this free.
Compassion within, so mote it be.

7. As you watch your paper burn down to ash, visualize all the guilt and pain you've been holding on to as a hazy black smoke swirling up into a ball in the center of yourself and lifting away from you into the sky. If safe to do so, allow the paper to burn out fully on its own. Thank the fire element for its aid. You may now extinguish your candle flames. Your work is now complete.

Healing Ancestral Trauma

Negative energies within build up over the years from childhood and before. Some traumas you're clutching may not even be your own, but passed down through your family for generations. While it's wonderful to honor and connect with ancestors, holding on to their past pain and trauma is not the way. It's time for you to take back your spirit, move past this vicious cycle, and rise up into your own power, leaving this past baggage behind. This pain is not your own and it's time to let it go.

Materials to Gather

- 1 stick thyme incense for honoring ancestors and purity
- Paper and pen

Steps to Take

1. Cleanse, ground, and center as needed.

2. Sit comfortably in a space that is personal to you where you feel safe and relax your mind.

3. Light your incense and say, "I light this incense to honor my ancestors and bring purity to my spirit."

4. Take your paper and pen and write down three negative patterns that you have noticed in your life that can be attributed to ancestral trauma.

5. Recite the following:

I thank my ancestors for their sacrifices.
I accept and acknowledge

*the experiences that hap-
pened before my time.
I accept and acknowledge
the residual negative energies
that have been passed down
throughout the years.
I release them from my spirit; it
is time to set them free.*

6. Now imagine these negative patterns as a gray smoke swirling up, starting from your toes, gathering all of this negativity as the smoke moves up and out the top of your head.

7. Sit quietly for a few moments with your eyes closed and focus on how much lighter and freer you now feel. Allow your incense to burn down fully.

The importance of trusting your inner voice cannot be emphasized enough. In today's world you may often silence what your intuition is trying to relay in order to act in the manner you believe you should—to conform to what is expected of you in society instead of trusting yourself.

When you are connected to your inner spirit and unconscious self, your intuition will become stronger, making it easier to hear what it is trying to relay. Your intuition can help you make decisions, keep you safe, and uncover hidden truths. Trusting your own intuition can quite simply change your life, your health, and your witchcraft practice.

Some people are incredibly intuitive, and others less so. Those who seem to be naturally intuitive have likely from a young age trusted themselves and listened to what the unconscious mind was telling them. To trust your intuition, you must learn to really listen to your inner self. Your intuition is yet another aspect of your inner magic that is sitting patiently, waiting to be developed. The rituals that follow will help you to do just that.

Awaken Your Intuition

To awaken your intuition, you must learn to trust yourself, hear yourself, and not push aside that inner voice when it tries to speak. Intuition that is ignored is eventually silenced, creating a divide within yourself. Perform this ritual during the waxing or full moon phases, an optimal time for spells related to personal growth and wisdom.

Materials to Gather

- 1–2 drops clary sage essential oil (properly diluted) for clarity and awareness
- 1 silver candle for intuition

Steps to Take

1. Cleanse, ground, and center as needed.

2. Choose a space that is quiet where you will not be disturbed and sit comfortably, place a drop

or two of the clary sage essential oil on your index finger, and anoint your candle with it. Run your finger up the sides and around the center until you are satisfied. Be sure to use only a small amount of oil.

3. Intuition and visualization are connected to the air element, so focus on your breath and bring yourself to a state of deep, steady breathing.

4. Now light your candle and focus your gaze on the flame. Notice how the air makes the flame dance and sway as it burns. Imagine a glittering silver sphere in the middle of your forehead expanding to allow your inner knowledge, voice, and light to open up and float to the surface. Allow your spirit to reach out and receive this energy. Stay in this visualization for at least 5 minutes. Let your mind wander and focus on any visions or messages that may be trying to reach you.

5. Once you finish with your visualization, recite the following:

Clear the fog and open the mind.
Inner knowledge there to find.
My voice, my spirit, wild and free.
Intuition awakened, so shall it be.

6. Give thanks to the air element for its gentle aid, take one final deep breath, and extinguish your flame.

Pendant to Trust Your Intuition

You should always be tuned in to your intuition. If that inner voice is trying to tell you something, be present and connected enough to hear it clearly. This pendant can help strengthen that connection. This type of witch's tool is especially useful if you're just learning to trust your intuition because it can make that voice easier to hear. Begin this ritual on a Monday, which is connected to the moon and psychic awareness.

Materials to Gather

- Bowl of water
- 1 silver candle for intuition
- 1 blue candle for spirituality awareness
- Clean cloth
- 1 tiger's eye, lapis lazuli, or labradorite stone with a bale so that it may fit on a necklace
- 1 silver chain to further strengthen intuition
- Pin or ritual knife

Steps to Take

1. Cleanse, ground, and center as needed.

2. Choose your workspace. If you don't have an altar, choose a space where you are able to leave your candles and bowl of water for a full week. Relax your thoughts. Bring your mind into a space that is open and free. Allow yourself to be in a balanced, neutral state.

3. Set up your supplies with your bowl of water in the center of your space, flanked by your candles on either side. Lay your clean cloth out flat in front of your bowl and place your stone and chain on top of it.

4. On the silver candle, carve the word "intuition" with your pin or knife and then light the candle. On the blue candle, carve the word "awareness" and then light that one.

5. Slide your stone onto your silver chain. Hold it out in front of you and say, "Sacred pendant, element of the earth, awaken me to my intuition."

6. Now gently dip the necklace into the water and place it back in front of the bowl. Say, "Flowing water, help my spirit to open up and listen."

7. Close your eyes, place both hands above the necklace, and recite the following:

I open my spirit and listen well.
Intuition awakened with this spell.
Always there to lead the way.
I trust in you come night, come day.

8. Open your eyes and thank the elements for their aid, then fold the sides of your cloth over the pendant.

9. Extinguish your candles and leave everything set just as it is. Each day at the same time you will repeat steps 5–7 for the next 6 days. Then on the following day, which will again be the Monday, you can begin to wear your newly charmed pendant.

Throughout the text I reference days of the week for the spells and rituals. Each day of the week has certain magical energies attached to it. Here is a brief overview:

- **Sunday:** success, strength, spirituality, healing, protection, creativity
- **Monday:** emotional healing, psychic awareness, intuition, wisdom, purification, dreams
- **Tuesday:** protection, courage, passion, marriage, energy
- **Wednesday:** divination, wisdom, change, communication
- **Thursday:** prosperity, abundance, money, health, loyalty, business, happiness
- **Friday:** love, fertility, friendship, harmony, growth, beauty, romance
- **Saturday:** hope, banishing, longevity, dreams, goals, protection

Intuitive Eating Exercise

The concept of intuitive eating is all about trusting yourself and your body. Eating in this manner will help free your spirit from any guilt or negative feelings surrounding food. Your body knows when it's hungry; it also knows what it requires to keep it strong and healthy. Only you know what your body needs based on how it's feeling and what it's saying. You just need to listen and learn to differentiate between real hunger and cravings.

Materials to Gather

- 1 blue candle for intuition
- Paper and a pen

Steps to Take

1. For a full 3 days you will listen closely and eat only when your body tells you it needs something, and then eat only what it tells you it is needing. Remember to pay attention and acknowledge when something is just a craving and not a true need.

2. Keep your paper, pen, and candle by your bedside if possible. At the start of each day before getting out of bed, light your candle, record your waking mood, and recite the following:

> Intuition within, guide me well.
> I shall learn to listen with this spell.

> Each day to feel and clearly see.
> As my will, so mote it be.

3. Extinguish your candle and begin your regular routine.

4. Throughout the day, each time you eat, record the time, what you ate, and how you were feeling. Remember to eat only when your body is telling you it needs something. At the end of each day, record your mood once again.

5. On the fourth day go through your 3-day food log. Notice any patterns that have arisen in the times, moods, and types of foods you ate. Consider how you can use this information to feed yourself better every day without worrying about counting calories or macros but by relying on your body to tell you what it needs. This is simply another way of connecting with your most inner self and following your intuition.

Crystal Charm Pouch to Awaken Psychic Abilities

We all have the ability to tap in to our psychic selves. Developing these skills will provide you with a heightened level of awareness within yourself and the universe, enabling you to be more in tune with, connected to, and mindful of the greater energies that surround you.

Materials to Gather

- 1 clear quartz stone for psychic abilities
- 1 amethyst stone for clairvoyance
- 1 celestite stone for attunement with higher realms
- 1 moonstone for insight
- 1–2 drops lemongrass essential oil for psychic development (properly diluted)
- 2 blue candles for spiritual awareness and intuition
- 1 purple pouch

Steps to Take

1. Cleanse, ground, and center as needed.

2. Sit comfortably in a calming, quiet space and relax your mind.

3. Place your crystals directly in front of you with the clear quartz in the center and the three other stones placed around to create a triangle. This positioning allows the crystals to feed off each other and work together to heighten their individual properties.

4. Now place the lemongrass essential oil on your index finger and anoint your two candles. You need not use much oil; just a little will do. Place the candles at the top of your space on either side of your crystal formation and light them.

5. Place both of your hands above your crystals, palms facing down, close your eyes, and recite the following:

Sacred crystals, open my mind.
Hidden knowledge I shall find.
Let me see what is not there.
By light, by dark, by earth and air.

6. Place the four crystals inside your pouch, tie it up, and say, "So mote it be." You may now extinguish your flames. Have this pouch with you whenever you are performing any divination practices or psychic meditations to assist in opening up your mind and heightening your sense of awareness.

Preparation Spell for Divination Work

Opening the spirit up with divination practices can be a powerful tool to enhance your overall wellness and magic. Deepening the connection with your higher self and the universal energies that surround you can provide a strong sense of self and confidence. This spell may be recited prior to any divination work to enhance your abilities, resulting in a more enriching experience.

Materials to Gather

- 1 purple candle for divination
- 2 labradorite stones for psychic abilities, awareness, and intuition

Steps to Take

1. Cleanse, ground, and center as needed.

2. Sit comfortably in a space where you feel relaxed and unburdened. Allow your mind to become clear and calm. Take three deep breaths and concentrate on breathing slow and steady.

3. Light your candle and hold one of your labradorite stones in each hand.

4. Stare just past your candle flame and recite the following three times:

My mind is open, light, and free. Intuition and insight, so mote it be.

5. Leave your candle burning (if safe to do so) and prepare your space as needed for the divination practice of your choice.

There are many types of divination practiced throughout the world. Divination can become a valuable tool for not only your magic but overall well-being. Some common divination methods used in the craft include tarot and oracle cards, scrying, reading tea leaves, pendulums, runes, and numerology. Do some research and try out some different methods to see which methods most align with your own practice.

Ritual to Recall Past Lives

The concept of reincarnation is a mysterious and intriguing one. Your soul is on a journey. The knowledge that with each new life you'll learn lessons and have experiences that make you wiser and more complete each time is powerful. Taking time to connect with and remember your past lives, even just bits and pieces, can feed your spirit and provide valuable insight into your witchcraft practice and the person you're becoming.

Materials to Gather

- 1 stick mugwort incense for psychic abilities
- 2 angel aura quartz stones for past-life recall (optional)
- 1 black tourmaline stone for protection

Steps to Take

1. Cleanse, ground, and center as needed.

2. Sit comfortably in the quietest space in your home, place your black tourmaline in front of you with the quartz on either side, if using, and light your incense. Take a moment to focus on your breathing, creating a relaxed space for your body, mind, and spirit. Maintaining a sense of ease throughout the process is essential to open the places inside yourself that must be accessed to receive these memories.

3. Close your eyes and visualize yourself in a beautifully green and vast forest. When you look in front of you in the distance, you can see a doorway adorned with leaves and colorful flowers guarded by a majestic white stag. This doorway is your destination. On the other side are the answers that you seek, the past-life memories that will enhance and enrich your present human experience.

4. Begin to make your way toward this magical doorway that you are so eager to walk through. Take each step with care, taking your time to fully see your journey in your mind's eye. Take notice of what kinds of trees

you are passing and if you pass any animals or certain flowers. Acknowledge the smells and sounds that are happening around you as you walk your path toward the doorway. See it getting closer with each step you take.

5. Once you reach the doorway, ask the stag for permission to enter; the stag is the keeper and will determine if your intentions are worthy of passing through. If he denies you, don't despair. You can refocus your mind and try again another day.

6. Once you do gain access and pass through over the threshold, accept and believe what you see. You may see only shapes, colors, or fuzzy outlines of objects when you are first beginning this journey. Recalling past lives

can take time, so do not rush the process. You will get there when the time is right.

7. Repeat this visualization as often as is needed to gain the insight you desire. Each time you begin, start your journey from the same place, though the journey toward the door will get faster each time as you already know your way and the stag will be there waiting to grant you access as he has already given you permission. Each time you pass through the door, your visions of what lies beyond will become clearer and more detailed. You may wish to record what you see each time as to not forget any important details. Relight your incense each time and replace as needed.

As a witch, you are connected to nature; it is a part of you, and the impact that nature has on your spirit is a profound one. Nature feeds your spirit and allows it to grow, feel free, and be strong. The more bonded and in tune with nature you feel, the more positive your outlook on life will be. You will be better able to deal with stressful situations when they arise, your immune system will be more equipped to fight off illness, and your magical practice will gain power and strength from nature's energy.

There are so many ways to add nature into your life: live seasonally; follow the cycles of the moon; grow your own food, herbs, or flowers; connect with the individual elements; and regularly give thanks or offerings to nature for her gifts. The following rituals will give you ways to make this connection strong and everlasting.

Bonding with Your Local Land

Making time each day to connect with nature will strengthen your craft, spirit, and overall wellness. Taking even 5 minutes a day to get outside, breathe in the fresh air, or give a short thanks to Mother Earth for her gifts will help to form this lifelong bond. This exercise is all about getting to know nature in your local area. Making a connection to your local land is an important step on the journey toward a spirit that is vibrant and whole.

Materials to Gather

- Outdoor space
- Camera

Steps to Take

1. Make sure you have your phone or a camera to take pictures and head out into your neighborhood. Walk the streets, visit a park, a nearby forest, or even your own backyard if you

have one. Choose three to five plants that you notice on your outing and take pictures of them.

2. Once you get back home, use an app or Internet search to identify the plants that you chose to take pictures of.

3. Once you have them identified, take time to research each one. Find out their history and any benefits, cautions, medicinal benefits, and magical properties that they hold.

4. Start a section in your journal or grimoire dedicated to local plant life and record your findings. Include pictures and any relevant information you come across in your research.

5. Repeat this process until you can identify all of the main local plant life in your area. This knowledge will show your commitment to the land on which you live as well as to Mother Nature as a whole.

6. Lastly, take time to go out and gather a leaf or flower from each plant, with permission from the plant of course. Bring them home and perform a simple blessing ritual for each one. Go through them at your own pace until you have worked your way through the complete list. Take your time with the process. It will likely take weeks or even months for you to make your way through all of the different plant life your area is blessed with. (Make sure you can identify poison oak and ivy before you start cutting and collecting!)

We are all nature witches. At the heart of every witch is nature and the elements. It can be no other way, for magic cannot exist without the energies of Mother Earth and the universe surrounding us, lifting us up, and giving us strength. The root of all magic truly is the land. Take time each day to remember and acknowledge this.

Full Moon Ritual to Connect with the Universe

Being connected to things greater than yourself is a spiritually enriching way to be. Connecting spirit to the energies that surround you, that can be felt but not seen, enables you to attain spiritual growth and appreciate the unseen things that many don't acknowledge. This creates a layer of fulfillment within, leading to a happier, healthier, and more powerful spirit.

Materials to Gather

- Bowl of soil to represent earth
- 1 stick incense of your choice to represent air
- 1 red candle to represent fire
- Chalice with drinking water to represent water

Steps to Take

1. Cleanse, ground, and center as needed.

2. Breathe deep and position yourself comfortably in your chosen space. Your altar is an ideal place for this if you have one. Set up your four elemental representations in the center of your space in a diamond shape. Place the soil to the north, incense to the east, candle to the south, and chalice to the west. These positions will symbolize the corresponding direction to each element.

3. First pick up your dish of soil, turn to the north, place one hand in the dish, and say, "I embrace earth." Place the dish back into its original position.

4. Next pick up your incense, turn east, light it, and say, "I embrace air." Place the incense back into its original position.

5. Then pick up your candle, turn south, light the wick, and say, "I embrace fire." Place the candle back into its original position.

6. Lastly, pick up your chalice, turn west, take a long drink of the water, and say, "I embrace water." Place the chalice back into its original position.

7. Now sit back at your space, bring your arms above your head, palms facing the sky, and say, "I open my heart and spirit to the magic of the universe and its energy."

8. Bring your arms down, close your eyes, and spend 5–10 minutes in silence with a calm and open mind. Allow your senses to access and react to all that surrounds you. Feel the energies in the air and enable your spirit to reach out and connect with those energies. Open your eyes and say, "So mote it be." Allow your candle and incense to burn down naturally if safe to do so.

Taking time to connect with each individual element will not only strengthen your connection to nature as a whole but will also deepen your relationships with each of the individual elements that allow you to sustain life. This will help you tap in to the properties and magical energies each element holds, enriching your spirit in new and exciting ways. Allow the earth to ground and nurture you, air to enhance intuition and bring knowledge, fire to purify and transform, and water to cleanse and heal. The elements are needed to sustain both your physical body and spiritual self.

There are many ways to connect with these elements in your daily life by taking simple and practical actions: Spend time outside, take a walk, and feel the earth beneath your feet; feel and appreciate the air on your face and filling your lungs with each breath; relish in the warmth of the sun on your skin or the beauty of a candle flame; properly hydrate yourself by drinking pure water or sit by a stream and take in the calming sounds of the flowing water. The following rituals will provide you with specific ways to connect with each of the four elements.

Ritual to Connect with Earth

The earth grounds you and provides stability. Earth is the element from which all life grows, and it is always there to nourish, strengthen, and care for you. It is wise to show your gratitude and take time to acknowledge and connect with her every day.

Materials to Gather	Steps to Take
• Outdoor space • An offering for Mother Earth	1. Begin this ritual by either taking a walk around your neighborhood and visiting a local park or forest if you are so lucky to live by one, or by spending time in your own backyard. Spend 15–20 minutes

in your chosen space feeling your feet on the ground; appreciating the beauty of the trees, plants, and birds; and being mindful and aware of all the sights, smells, and sounds that surround you.

2. While you are exploring your outdoor space, choose a natural object to leave as an offering to nature. This could be a fallen acorn, pine cone, flower, leaf, or special rock you find. Be sure to take only things that are allowed and have naturally fallen to the ground. When you find the right object, pick it up and thank the earth for this gift.

3. Next find a tree, any tree that calls out to you on your outing, such as a tree in the park, your yard, a forest, or wherever you are spending this time. Stand by the tree and leave your offering on the ground in front of it. Recite the following (this can be in your head if you do not have privacy):

Sacred Earth Mother, this gift I share.
To show my thanks for your love and care.
I commit to always honor you.
From roots to sky, it shall remain true.

4. Spend a few minutes sitting with your tree before you finish. You may return to this same tree and leave offerings regularly if you wish.

-€€€-

Ritual to Connect with Air

Air is an element that is surrounding you and within you at every moment of the day. The air is the breath that fills your lungs, the cool breeze on a hot summer day, or a moving piece of music. Embracing this element will allow you to feel freedom, awaken your intuition, and ignite the wisdom held within.

Materials to Gather

- Outdoor space (you may do this by a window if necessary)
- A blanket
- 2 lapis lazuli stones for air connection

Steps to Take

1. Find a space outside where you are comfortable and lie down on your blanket. Or make yourself comfortable at the best window

in your home if you are unable to be outside. Hold one lapis lazuli stone in each hand.

2. Spend a few moments relaxing and focusing on your breath. Concentrate on deep, slow, and steady breaths. You are already connected to air with every breath you take; in this moment be mindful and conscious of the process.

3. Now stare up at the sky and appreciate the color, the depth,

and the vastness of it all. Focus on the clouds and their movement patterns and shapes. Spend some time using your imagination as you may have done as a child and find animals, stories, and magic in the formations of the clouds.

4. When you feel finished, say, "Beautiful element of air, I honor you and appreciate your magic and blessings." Stay in your space until you feel ready to go.

Ritual to Connect with Fire

Fire is the most volatile of the elements and should be handled with care, but it also holds incredible power when you take proper time to connect with and embrace it. Fire represents light and beautiful transformation. Utilize this energy to ignite passion within yourself, create powerful change, and to summon forth the courage you have within yourself.

Materials to Gather

- 2 red candles to represent fire
- 1 gold or yellow candle to represent the sun

Steps to Take

1. Clear your mind and make yourself comfortable. Place your candles in front of you in a line with the gold/yellow one in the center.

2. Light each of the red candles and then say, "Fire element, I honor you." Now light your gold/yellow candle and state, "Life-giving Sun, I honor you."

3. Now sit back, relax, and focus your gaze on the warm light of the flames. Position your palms toward the candles and feel the warmth nourishing them. Be careful not to be so close that it gets too hot or you risk burning yourself.

4. Focus your mind on the life-giving heat and energy that is emitting from the candlelight. Allow yourself to feel passion, vitality, and strength within you. Concentrate on feeling these powerful fire-driven energies flowing freely. Stay in this state for at least 10 minutes. When you feel the ritual is complete, give thanks to the fire element and extinguish your flames.

Ritual to Connect with Water

Water rises, falls, and flows with a beautiful and majestic ease. Water brings energies that cleanse, heal, and ignite love. Listen to the rain, have a relaxing bath, hydrate yourself, and let these energies wash over you. Embrace the water element and allow it to bring happiness, health, and harmony to your spirit and life.

Materials to Gather

- Rainwater
- Bowl
- 3 aquamarine stones
- Towel

Steps to Take

1. First you will need rainwater. The next time it is going to rain, place a cup or bowl outside and leave it until it is full or it stops raining.

2. Collect your water and transfer it to a clean bowl on your altar or workspace.

3. Next place your aquamarine stones around your bowl in the shape of an upside-down triangle (the symbol for water).

4. Place your hands into the water, move them around, and wiggle your fingers. Feel the cool and wet sensations on your skin. Allow your spirit to take on the properties of the water element: happiness, love, cleansing, and harmony. Feel these things flowing in and around yourself, feeling lighter and freer with each passing moment. Water is soothing and uplifting; concentrate on taking these properties into your spirit.

5. Remove your hands from the water and let them hover, palms down, just above the bowl. Recite the following:

> Sacred water, wild and free.
> I honor you from river to sea.
> Ebbing, flowing, to love and heal.
> My gratitude and thanks be revealed.

6. Dry your hands and thank the water element once more for its service.

Balancing the spiritual energies within yourself will allow for the proper flow of vibrations within your whole self. Chapter 2 discussed the importance of balancing energies within the home, and the energies housed within yourself are no different. When energies within are unbalanced, this leads to blockages that do not allow things to properly flow, which can lead to erratic emotions and a sense of unhappiness and cause you to build spiritual walls around yourself for protection.

It is easier to feel balanced when things in life are going smoothly, but to experience true inner balance is to maintain this state when life becomes challenging. It is important for us to regularly perform grounding and centering rituals, deal with past pains, take time-outs, meditate, and do things that bring us joy in order to attain this balanced spirit on a regular basis. The following rituals will help you to bring your energies into balance and keep them there in your daily life, regardless of what life might throw at you.

Essential Grounding Ritual for Balance

Performing a grounding sequence is meant to bring your energies into a balanced and present state via connection with the earth. Incorporating grounding regularly will have a positive impact on your spirit, as well as elevate the work you do in your witchcraft practice.

It's good practice to ground yourself before, and sometimes after, any magical work. Many of the rituals within these pages will suggest this. This ritual takes only a couple of minutes and you can do it almost anywhere. It's optimal if you're able to perform this outside. You may also choose to cast a circle before beginning to purify and protect the space. Aim to complete this once per day at a time most convenient to you for optimal benefits.

Materials to Gather

- Yourself

Steps to Take

1. Find a space where you feel relaxed. If you're indoors, choosing a spot by your favorite window, some fresh flowers, or a plant to have an extra nature connection present would be perfect.

2. Stand barefoot, close your eyes, take a couple of deep breaths, and press both feet down firmly. Feel every inch of them connecting with the surface beneath.

3. Visualize now that you're growing roots into the earth from your feet, providing you with an anchor and stability. Perhaps you're a wise old oak tree or a beautiful flower.

4. Imagine the energy being pulled up from your roots and moving evenly throughout your body. Feel it extending up from your feet, into your core, to the tips of your fingers, and the top of your head until you feel a sense of balance within. Utilize the earth's energy in this moment; let it replenish you or absorb any excess energy you may be carrying.

5. Take a couple more deep breaths here and recite the following:

> *I am grounded. I am present. I am magic.*

6. Open your eyes, wiggle your toes, wrap your arms around yourself in a gentle hug, release one final exhale, and bring your arms down to your sides. Give your body a little stretch and thank the earth for its service.

Vital Centering Ritual

It is good practice to take a moment to center yourself prior to completing your magical work, which is suggested throughout our rituals here, as well as anytime you are feeling off or out of sorts. Centering brings your spirit back into alignment, eases anxiety, and brings a sense of calm and clarity to self. Without attaining that feeling of centered balance, your spirit can become depleted from the excess energies swirling within. The more you complete this exercise, the easier it will be to attain this centered state of being.

Materials to Gather

* Yourself

Steps to Take

1. Stand or sit comfortably in your chosen space. This practice is easy enough that it can really be performed wherever and whenever you feel it's needed. Close your eyes and take three to five long, deep breaths; really focus on your breathing and stretch out the length of time it takes you to complete one full inhale and exhale.

2. Do a quick body scan. Feel your toes, legs, arms, hands, and every part of yourself all the way to the top of your head. Notice where you feel tense and where you may be holding excess energy.

3. Bring your focus to your center. Now imagine all of that energy being gathered up into a brilliant ball of white light in your core. Visualize strings of that light moving back out slowly and evenly throughout yourself. This is allowing the energy to become balanced and neutral.

4. Bring your focus back to the white energy ball in your core, now a little smaller but still there anchoring your energies to your center.

5. Open your eyes and say, aloud or in your mind, "My spirit is centered, my mind at ease, my body balanced."

Casting a circle prior to your magical work is a personal choice of every witch and not at all mandatory. Common times to do this include during more lengthy rituals or when extra protection is needed in your space, though some choose to cast a circle every time they practice. Some easy ways to do this with the proper focused intention include visualization, using your athame or wand to mark your circle, or creating a physical circle with a magical object such as crystals.

Ritual to Move Stagnant Energies

Your spirit can at times feel stuck, stilted, or in limbo. You reach a certain point in your spiritual journey and then plateau, like the energies have nowhere else to travel. This ritual will assist in enabling your energies to flow and move freely once again so that you may continue to evolve and develop your spiritual practice.

Materials to Gather

- 2 drops eucalyptus essential oil (properly diluted) for growth
- 1 carnelian stone for energy and motivation
- 1 rose quartz stone for cleansing and healing

Steps to Take

1. Prepare yourself for a brisk walk or run. Wear something that makes you feel confident and comfortable.

2. Bring yourself into a centered and grounded state.

3. Anoint each wrist with a drop of eucalyptus essential oil and say, "Sacred eucalyptus, allow my energies to move free and grow with me."

4. Now place your stones, one in each pocket, and say, "Carnelian, provide me with energy and motivation. Rose quartz, allow me to cleanse and heal."

5. Head outside into the wild and focus on your steps, your muscles working, and your breath. If you choose to walk, make sure your pace is quick enough to work up a sweat.

6. Visualize any unmoving energies beginning to swirl around and pick up steam. See these energies as colors of the rainbow.

There can be many different energies within that have gotten stuck. See these energies begin to move and flow free, branching out evenly within yourself. Make your outing at least 15–20 minutes.

7. When you arrive back home, take a long and leisurely shower. This will allow any negative energies that may have been uprooted to be washed away, leaving you with cleansed and balanced energies to take on whatever the coming days may bring.

Craft a Dream Box to Recharge the Spirit

Your spirit may become broken or saddened or lose its sense of life and vitality. This occurs especially when you're too busy to take the proper time to nourish this part of yourself. The following ritual is a simple way to recharge those spiritual batteries. The new moon, a time for renewal and recharging, is optimal for this ritual.

Materials to Gather

- 1 red candle for strength and passion
- Small decorative box
- Items to represent your current most important dreams
- 1 each of moonstone, tiger's eye, and rose quartz stones for creativity and focus
- 3 drops sweet orange oil for prosperity and success

Steps to Take

1. Cleanse, ground, and center as needed.

2. Gather your materials and sit comfortably in your space. Light your candle and focus your mind on your dream life. Be specific in the details. Taking time to envision your dreams can breathe new life into your spirit and get those positive energies flowing.

3. Take your box and begin adding in your items that represent your dreams. As you do this, visualize what your life will look like when they come to fruition. How will your spirit feel once these dreams become your reality?

4. Place your three crystals on top, add the drops of oil, and close the box.

5. Now take the box and hold it above your candle flame to charge the box with passionate transformation energies to help your dreams manifest. Be careful it is a safe distance above the flame. As you do this, recite the following:

Spirit within I breathe new life.
Rejuvenated and free from any strife.
Passionate dreams, planted like a tree.
This is my will, so mote it be.

6. You may now extinguish your flame. Place the box on your dresser or altar and each morning, place your hands atop the box and say, "My spirit is charged and ready to help manifest my dreams."

7. You may repeat this ritual or update your box whenever your dreams shift direction.

The new moon is the phase of the moon where it is just beginning its journey on the way to being bright and full. This makes the energy at this time in the moon's cycle perfect for performing magic related to renewal and recharging, setting fresh intentions, health, confidence, and money. Mark the new moons on your calendar so you never miss a chance to tap in to this fresh new energy.

Being present and practicing mindfulness daily is one of the best ways to strengthen your connection to spirit and your wellness as a whole. Being mindful is having awareness of your own actions, being present in each moment, thinking of others in your life, and considering your actions on the environment and on your own senses and feelings. It is being conscious of and in tune with yourself, those around you, and the planet.

Being mindful in each moment will not only mean your life will be more fulfilling and meaningful, but it will also give you insights into other people and the world around you. It will help you gain wisdom of your inner self, what's truly important to you, and what is the best path for you to be on at this time. It will also open your mind up to your witchcraft practice and what elements to focus on and work with to get the most out of your magical work.

Walking Meditation for Mindfulness

Walking meditations are a great companion to traditional meditations, working well for those who have trouble maintaining focus during seated meditations. They're a great way to tune in to surrounding magic and cherish being in the moment.

Materials to Gather

- 1 clear quartz stone for awareness
- 1 hematite stone for connection to spirit

Steps to Take

1. Cleanse, ground, and center as needed.

2. Relax your mind and choose your walking route. Choose something familiar and plan it out so you're not making decisions about direction during the meditation portion.

3. Carry your stones, one in each hand. This will allow the stones to be charged with positive energies of gratitude and appreciation throughout your walk as well as enable you to absorb the properties of awareness and connection throughout the walk.

4. As you begin to move, focus on getting a steady rhythm with your breath and pace. Check in with yourself and acknowledge how your body is feeling. Notice any sensations, areas that are tense, and those that feel more relaxed.

5. Move your concentration to your legs and feet. Feel your muscles working and feet connecting to the ground with each step you take. Appreciate your body and all of the amazing things it does for you each day.

6. Now take in your surroundings. Be present in each moment throughout your walk and notice the smells, colors, sights, and sounds that you are passing by. Let the appreciation for life, nature, and all of their gifts feed your spirit.

7. Once you arrive back home, either sit on your steps or in your house for just a few minutes before doing anything else. While your mind is still relaxed and at ease from the meditation, mentally make a list of everything that you are feeling appreciation for in this moment and allow your spirit to truly embrace the joy that these things bring.

Gratitude Ritual

Expressing gratitude in your daily life for things both large and small is an integral part of living mindfully. Being aware and acknowledging all the universe has blessed you with is crucial for a spirit that feels complete and a magical practice that yields positive results. You may perform this ritual each day as part of your spiritual practice.

Materials to Gather

- 1 silver or white candle for gratitude and blessings
- Piece of paper and a pen
- Small Mason jar or decorative box

Steps to Take

1. Cleanse, ground, and center as needed.

2. Choose a space where you can leave your candle and jar set up. Arrange your items to your liking, clear your mind, and focus your thoughts toward feelings of gratitude and thankfulness.

3. Light your candle. Now take your paper and pen and write three things that you feel grateful for in this moment.

4. Once they are written, recite them out loud or in your mind, then fold your paper into three.

5. Hold the paper in your palms and recite the following:

> *Universe, I am grateful.*
> *Universe, I am blessed.*
> *I am eternally thankful.*
> *For each gift I have professed.*

6. Place the paper in your jar and put on the lid. You may now extinguish your flame. Repeat this same ritual each day. You may visit your jar and reread some of your entries whenever you need a reminder that you have much to be thankful for.

Ritual for Welcoming Positivity

Your spirit, health, and magic will thrive in a positive environment. Negativity can dampen and drag down your spirit when it's meant to shine. This ritual allows you to welcome more positive energy and release some of the negative.

Materials to Gather

- 1 gold votive candle for positivity
- Small pot filled with soil
- Happy music
- Piece of paper and a pen
- 3 stones of your choosing

Steps to Take

1. Cleanse, ground, and center as needed.

2. Choose a room where you will have some space and privacy. Place your candle on a table with your pot of soil, or on the floor if it's safe to do so, in the center of the room. Start to play your chosen music.

3. Sit in front of your candle and light it.

4. Take your paper and pen and make a list of all the positive words you can think of (e.g., "happiness," "joy," "travel," "health," "love,"

"success"); write down everything you can think of that will bring positivity to your spirit and help to keep it in a positive place.

5. Now gently place your paper under the candle so that it catches the wax.

6. Stand for just a minute or two and dance around your candle. Please take extra care when doing this step and keep a safe distance to not knock your candle over. You may do this step for as long as you wish. While you dance, allow yourself to let the music feed your spirit waves of positive energy. Feel the happiness and uplifting energy deep within yourself.

7. Once you have finished with your dance, take your paper and fold it in three, making sure to leave any drips of wax on the paper.

8. Take your paper and bury it in the soil.

9. Now take your three stones and place them in a triangle shape on top of the soil. Place your hands above the pot and recite the following:

Positivity in spirit and in mind.
Negative energy is left behind.
My spirit light and finally free.
As my will, so mote it be.

10. Extinguish your flame, or let it burn down naturally if safe to do so. Place your positivity pot in the most central room of your home where you will most often be able to align with the positive energy it has been imbued with.

Sigil to Open Your Heart

Sigils are a design or symbol created with a specific intention in mind. The most powerful sigil magic occurs when you've crafted one yourself. They don't need to be fancy and there is no need to be an artist to create one. This sigil practice will focus on opening your heart to the magic of life and relationships.

Materials to Gather

- 1 pink candle to represent love
- Piece of paper
- Pink pen or marker

Steps to Take

1. Cleanse, ground, and center as needed.

2. Choose a space in your home you feel a connection with, clear your mind, and light your candle.

3. For this exercise you will craft a permanent sigil, meaning it is meant to last. Opening your heart to love is an intention that will not change and may sometimes need help to stay open.

4. State your intention out loud, "My heart is open and accepting."

5. Draw your sigil. To draw the sigil, you may gain inspiration from symbols associated with your intention, such as a heart in this instance. You may also use the letters in the associated word, in this case "heart." This is generally done using each letter in the word only once and omitting the vowels. So you may use the letters *H*, *R*, and *T* and a heart to create your sigil. Arrange the letters in

an abstract way so that it is not obvious right away what they are. You will know. Be creative and make the sigil pleasing to your eye.

6. Lastly, you will charge your sigil. There are many ways to do this, but for today you will hold your open palms above your sigil and visualize a brilliant pink light emanating from your palms and transferring energy of openness, love, and acceptance into the sigil. Ensure your spirit is in a good place while you do this.

7. With your palms still in place and holding your visualization, recite the following:

My heart is open, my heart is free.
Love and acceptance, so mote it be.

8. Now imagine the pink light emptying from your hands and into the sigil. Your sigil is now charged. You may now extinguish your flame.

9. Place the sigil on your altar or in an intimate space of your home such as your bedroom. You may wish to recharge your sigil periodically as you feel it's needed.

Witch Jar for Receiving Abundance

The abundance referenced here is abundance of spirit: to live full of joy, light, and strength; to live in the moment; to nurture and cherish oneself; and to feed your spirit well. The following spell jar will help you remember that you deserve a life of rich nonmaterialistic abundance and prosperity.

Materials to Gather

- Small Mason jar with lid
- 1 white candle for spiritual connection
- 1 blue candle for spiritual awareness
- 3 tablespoons dried basil for abundance and spiritual growth
- 1 amethyst stone for wisdom
- 1 carnelian stone for confidence
- 1 citrine stone for success
- 3 drops cinnamon essential oil for abundance and prosperity
- 1 white ribbon to represent your spirit

Steps to Take

1. Cleanse, ground, and center as needed.

2. Sit comfortably in your workspace and direct your thoughts toward feelings of abundance.

3. Place your Mason jar in the middle of your space with one candle on either side.

4. Light your candles. While you do this, focus on the spiritual abundance that you already have in your life and how you might open yourself to accept more. Allow yourself to feel love, positivity, and peace. What aspects of spiritual abundance do you not allow yourself to have more of? Maybe you have trouble staying positive or showing yourself some love. You deserve these things and so much more; remember this as you fill your jar.

5. First add the dried basil into the jar, then your crystals, and then the essential oil. While you're filling your jar, keep these energies of abundance within yourself. Feel optimistic and kind.

6. Lastly, tie the ends of your white ribbon together so that it forms a circle. This circle represents your continuous and complete spirit. Place the ribbon inside the jar and close the lid.

7. Place both hands above the jar, close your eyes, and recite the following three times:

Abundance is all around me. I devote to reaching out and embracing it fully.

8. You may now extinguish your flames and place the jar on your altar or other place of prominence as a reminder that your life can be as spiritually abundant as you allow it to be.

As part of any magical wellness journey, you must let yourself be still. You must accept that you are not a machine, that you need rest, and that it's perfectly okay to sit and enjoy just being with yourself. There are many things we can do to embrace stillness, such as doing a meditation, sitting quietly with a tea or coffee, or watching the rain out the window.

It is in these moments of stillness when we can become more attune with our own spirit and with the universe. This is the place that fosters creativity, eases stress, and allows your magic to flow. In a world where there is so much noise, you must take these moments to step back and just breathe. Breathe, gain insight, tap in to your intuition, and bring the body into a state of balance. Incredibly magical things can happen within you when you are doing nothing at all.

Meditation to Welcome Stillness

You must get comfortable with just being. The moments when you are just being still are the moments that connect you to your spirit and the universe. These are the moments where you train yourself to be mindful and present in your daily life. This meditation is all about embracing the quiet and allowing yourself this time of stillness.

Materials to Gather

- 1 stick frankincense for meditation encouragement

Steps to Take

1. Cleanse, ground, and center as needed.

2. Choose a quiet space where you will not be disturbed, relax your mind, and light your incense.

3. Sit comfortably and close your eyes. Take five deep breaths and concentrate on making them slow, deep, and steady. Now focus on clearing your mind. You have nothing you need to think of now. Just keep focusing on your breathing.

4. It can be difficult to clear your mind of thoughts, so it may help to focus on seeing a single color

in your mind until you get enough practice keeping your thoughts clear. It will get easier the more you practice. If thoughts do arise during your practice, simply acknowledge them and let them go, then continue on with your practice. This is perfectly okay and is no cause for feelings of guilt or failure.

5. Stay in your meditation for 5 minutes. You are free to stay as long as you like, but if you're new to meditation, then beginning with 5 minutes and working your way up to longer amounts of time is a good starting point. Allow your incense to burn down fully if it hasn't already.

-⟨⟨⟨-

Ritual to Slow Down

Taking time to slow down and just let yourself be will ease stress, clear your mind, provide new perspective, and allow your spirit to feel content. You will be more productive in your life, and witchcraft practice, and your spirit will have time to recharge. This ritual helps you to relax and take a few moments to enjoy doing nothing and not worry about work or to-do lists.

Materials to Gather

- Chamomile tea to calm the mind
- 1 blue candle for peace
- 1 stick chamomile incense for harmony

Steps to Take

1. Cleanse, ground, and center as needed.

2. Make your tea and choose a space where you can sit quietly and not be disturbed.

3. Arrange your candle and incense in your space. Light your candle and say, "Blue candle flame, bring peace to my spirit." Next light your incense and say, "Sacred chamomile, bring harmony to my spirit."

4. Sit comfortably and begin to sip your tea. With your first five to ten sips state an affirmation that aligns with quieting your spirit and allowing it to simply be, such as, "My spirit is light" or "My spirit deserves time to recharge."

5. Continue to sip your tea in silence, focus on your breathing, close your eyes if you wish, and try not to allow any stressful thoughts to invade your tranquility. Take a moment to reflect on how you have been nourishing your spirit and giving it the attention it deserves. Let yourself feel good about this time you are providing for yourself. Try to spend at least 20 minutes in this space of still and quietness. Allow your candle and incense to burn down fully if you wish.

Spell for Accepting Your Limits

You may tend to take on too much and try to please everyone with little thought to your own well-being. You must be okay with taking time to recognize and accept your limits. When you've reached them, grant yourself permission to say no to things and do less. This ritual is about accepting yourself and knowing when your spirit needs a break.

Materials to Gather

- 3 drops eucalyptus essential oil for growth
- 2 drops lemongrass essential oil for positivity
- 1 drop peppermint essential oil for healing
- 1 hematite stone for grounding and calm
- 1 lapis lazuli stone for balance and spirituality

Steps to Take

1. Cleanse, ground, and center as needed.

2. Gather your materials and choose a diffuser method.

3. Set your intentions for your oil blend clear in your mind. Visualize yourself resting, taking on only as much as you can handle, and having extra time to focus on yourself. Keep this picture in your mind while you blend.

4. Add each oil one at a time into your diffuser and recite the following:

> I will no longer take on too much.
> I will accept my limits.
> I will only take on what works for me.
> I will allow my spirit to rest and heal.

5. Spend a moment appreciating the scents. Let the oils spread their magic throughout your space. Tune in to your spirit and feel the vibrations within becoming less burdened, more relaxed, and freer.

6. Now sit in the center of your space, holding one stone in each hand, close your eyes and just breathe. Focus your thoughts on this new commitment to yourself to be there for your own spirit, to feel positive about taking on less, and to imagine your extra responsibilities lifting from your shoulders and dissolving into the ether.

These journal prompts and affirmations are designed to keep you mindful and connected to spirit even, and perhaps especially, in times that are challenging when it may be easier for you to lose sight of the connection you have worked so diligently to build.

Journal Prompts for Spiritual Wellness

1. In this moment, how connected do you feel to your spiritual self?

2. What made you excited to get out of bed this morning?

3. Are there any darker parts of yourself that you have yet to face?

4. What are three things you can do each day to nurture your spiritual self?

5. Are you living your most authentic life? If not, what changes might you make so that your life is more in tune with your authentic self?

Daily Affirmations for Spiritual Wellness

- I am at peace.

- I am a magical being.

- My spirit is aligned with the universe.

- My spirit is complete and powerful.

- The light within me shall never dim.

Bibliography

Auryn, Mat. *Psychic Witch: A Metaphysical Guide to Meditation, Magick, & Manifestation*. Woodbury, MN: Llewellyn, 2020.

Beyerl, Paul. *The Master Book of Herbalism*. Custer, WA: Phoenix, 1984.

Blake, Deborah. *Everyday Witchcraft: Making Time for Spirit in a Too-Busy World*. Woodbury, MN: Llewellyn, 2015.

Chopra, Deepak. *Metahuman: Unleashing Your Infinite Potential*. New York: Harmony Books, 2019.

Colbin, Annemarie. *Food and Healing: How What You Eat Determines Your Health, Your Well-Being, and the Quality of Your Life*. 10th Anniversary Edition. New York: Ballantine Books, 1996.

Cunningham, Scott. *Cunningham's Encyclopedia of Wicca in the Kitchen*. 3rd ed. St. Paul, MN: Llewellyn, 2003.

Cunningham, Scott and David Harrington. *The Magical Household: Spells & Rituals for the Home*. Illustrated ed. St. Paul, MN: Llewellyn, 2002.

Ehrenreich, Barbara and Deirdre English. *Witches, Midwives & Nurses: A History of Women Healers*. 2nd ed. New York: Feminist Press, 2010.

Essential Oils: Natural Healing for Body and Soul. Morton Grove, IL: Publications International, 2018.

Franklin, Anna. *The Hearth Witch's Compendium: Magical and Natural Living for Every Day*. Woodbury, MN: Llewellyn, 2017.

Gilbert, Karen. *Natural Beauty: 35 Step-by-Step Projects for Homemade Beauty*. New York: CICO Books, 2013.

Greenleaf, Cerridwen. *The Book of Kitchen Witchery: Spells, Recipes, and Rituals for Magical Meals, an Enchanted Garden, and a Happy Home*. New York: CICO Books, 2016.

Hall, Judy. *The Crystal Bible: A Definitive Guide to Crystals*. Cincinnati: Walking Stick Press, 2003.

Holford, Patrick. *Optimum Nutrition for the Mind: Optimum Living Made Easy*. London, UK: Piatkus, 2007.

Miller, Daphne M.D. *Farmacology: Total Health from the Ground Up*. New York: William Morrow, 2013.

Murphy-Hiscock, Arin. *The House Witch: Your Complete Guide to Creating a Magical Space with Rituals and Spells for Hearth and Home*. Avon, MA: Adams Media, 2018.

Murphy-Hiscock, Arin. *The Witch's Book of Self-Care: Magical Ways to Pamper, Soothe, and Care for Your Body and Spirit*. Avon, MA: Adams Media, 2018.

Rider, Elizabeth. *The Health Habit: 7 Easy Steps to Reach Your Goals and Dramatically Improve Your Life*. Illustrated ed. Carlsbad, CA: Hay House, 2019.

Starhawk. *The Earth Path: Grounding Your Spirit in the Rhythms of Nature*. New York: HarperSanFrancisco, 2005.

Starhawk. *The Spiral Dance: A Rebirth of the Ancient Religion of the Great Goddess*. 20th Anniversary Edition. New York: HarperSanFrancisco, 1999.

Whitehurst, Tess. *Magical Housekeeping: Simple Charms & Practical Tips for Creating a Harmonious Home*. Woodbury, MN: Llewellyn, 2010.

Yardley, Katolen. *The Good Living Guide to Natural and Herbal Remedies: Simple Salves, Teas, Tinctures, and More*. New York: Good Books, 2016.

Index of Physical Ailments

Note: Page numbers in *italics* indicate rituals, recipes/formulas, crafts, and potions.

General Index

hair rinse for revitalization, *132–33*
rosemary cuticle oil, *131*
soothing hand salve for dry skin, *129*
sunburn soothing mist, *130*
witch's water for acne, *127*
Herbs. *See also* specific herbs
about: magical and wellness properties by
herb, 30–31; uses and benefits, 29, 30–31
Herb sachets, 78–81
about: for home, 78
building peaceful home, *80–81*
creating loving home, *79–80*
enhancing positive energies, *78–79*
spell sachet to overcome addiction, *157*
Hibiscus, magical and wellness
properties, 30–31
Home. *See also* Cleansing the home;
Energies in home, balancing; Environment, magical; Prosperity and abundance; Protecting the home
essential oil magic for, 82–85
herb sachets for, 78–81
magical mists for, 73–77
Hormone balance, 33, *116–17*, *174–75*.
See also Stress and anxiety, relieving
Hydration and water element, *92–93*

I

Immunity, boosting, 31, 33, 35, *123*. *See
also* Physical wellness
Inflammation, relieving, 31, 35, 117
Influenza. *See* Colds, coughs, and flu
Insomnia. *See* Sleep and dreams
Intuition
about: letting it guide you, 209
awakening, *209–10*
crystal charm pouch to awaken psychic
abilities, *214*
intuitive eating exercise, *213*
pendant to trust, *211–12*
recalling past lives, *216–17*

J

Journal
about: starting grimoire or, 27–28
accessing your shadow self, *204–5*
mental awareness prompts and
affirmations, 191
physical wellness prompts and
affirmations, 139
ritual for self-discovery, *183–84*
spiritual prompts and affirmations, 244

L

Labradorite, magical and wellness prop-
erties, 32–33
Lactation, stimulating, 31
Land (local), bonding with, *218–19*
Lapis lazuli, magical and wellness
properties, 32–33
Lavender, magical and wellness
properties, 30–31
Lemon balm, magical and wellness
properties, 30–31
Lemongrass oil, magical and wellness
properties, 34–35
Letting go of material possessions, *46–47*
Limits, spell for accepting, *242–43*
Liver health. *See* Detoxification
Love
Dark Chocolate Peanut Butter Energy
Balls for, *100–101*
herb sachet for creating loving home, *79–80*
self-love spell jar, *147–48* (*See also*
Self-acceptance)

M

Magic
body, mind, spirit and, 21–23
importance of nutrition for, 94 (*See also*
Nutrition and recipes)
ritual to connect inner magic, 22–23
Magical wellness
about: overview and perspective on,
12–13, 17; this book and, 15

about: witches and nature, 219
bonding with local land, *218–19*
full moon ritual to connect with the universe, *220–21*
Nausea, reducing, 31, 35, *114–15*
Neroli oil, magical and wellness properties, 34–35
Nervousness, 31, 33, 35. *See also* Stress and anxiety, relieving
Nettle, magical and wellness properties, 30–31
Nutrition and recipes, 94–107
about: eating intuitively, *213*; importance of nutrition for magic, 94; recipes, 95–107
Blueberry Bran Muffins for Grounding, *97–98*
"Cheesy" Lentil Pasta Bake for Peace and Purity, *106–7*
Cinnamon Cacao Granola for Prosperity, *99*
Dark Chocolate Peanut Butter Energy Balls for Love, *100–101*
Gut-Repairing Turmeric Latte, *124–25*
Immunity-Boosting Wellness Shot, *123*
Lemon Tahini Salad Dressing for Protection, *102*
Morning Magic Green Smoothie for Success, *95–96*
Mushroom and Greens Miso Stir-Fry for Psychic Abilities, *104–5*
Nourishing Hormone Smoothie, *174–75*
Three-Bean Salad for Abundance, *103*

O
Orange, qualities associated with, 37

P
Pain, relieving, 31, 33, 35, *117–18*, *122*. *See also* Headaches
Past lives, ritual to recall, *216–17*

Patchouli oil, magical and wellness properties, 34–35
Peace
"Cheesy" Lentil Pasta Bake for Peace and Purity, *106–7*
herb sachet for building peaceful home, *80–81*
Pendants, *175–76*, *211–12*
Peppermint, magical and wellness properties, 30–31
Peridot, magical and wellness properties, 32–33
Physical wellness. *See also* Herbal potions references; Nutrition and recipes; Index of Physical Ailments
about: connection between movement and magic, 90–91; hydration importance, 92; journal prompts and affirmations, 139
connect with water element, *92–93*
morning ritual to boost energy, *90–91*
tuning into your physical self, *88–89*
Pine oil, magical and wellness properties, 34–35
Pink, qualities associated with, 37
Plant blessing ritual, *44–45*
Playfulness essential oil blend, *83*
PMS, easing, 33
Positivity, ritual for welcoming, *236–37*
Pouch, lavender dream, *110*
Pouches, crystal. *See* Crystal pouches
Prosperity and abundance
about: manifesting in the home, 65
Cinnamon Cacao Granola for Prosperity, *99*
crystal pouch for boosting, *70–71*
drawing money into the home, *66–67*
gratitude ritual for, *67–68*
manifesting a prosperous home, *65–66*
Three-Bean Salad for Abundance, *103*
witch jar for receiving abundance (spiritual), *238–39*

full moon bath to embrace divine feminine within, *201–2*
full moon ritual to connect with the universe, *220–21*
healing ancestral trauma, *207–8*
journaling to access your shadow self, *204–5*
meditation for inner peace, *200–201*
meditation to find your true purpose, *196–97*
meditation to welcome stillness, *240–41*
presenting an offering to a deity, *203–4*
releasing guilt and gaining forgiveness, *206–7*
ritual to slow down, *241–42*
spell collage to connect with your authentic self, *194–96*
spell for accepting your limits, *242–43*
spell jar to access inner wisdom, *199–200*
Stress and anxiety, relieving, *160–68*
about (*See also* Spiritual wellness): crystals for, 33; essential oil for, 35; herbs for, 31; mental/emotional wellness and, 141; positive relationships and, 180
calming ritual salt bath, *164–65*
candle ritual for combatting stress, *163*
five-minute ritual for easing anxiety, *160–61*
relaxation magical mist, *74*
relaxation meditation with crystals, *165–66*
spell jar to alleviate worry, *161–62*
sunset ritual to ease depression symptoms, *166–68*
Sunburn, soothing, *130*
Sweet orange oil, magical and wellness properties, 34–35
T
Teas, magical, 134–38
about: benefits and brewing, 134–35
Carob Lavender Blend to Banish Cravings, *136*

Cinnamon Cardamom Blend to Balance Blood Sugar, *135*
Hibiscus Blend to Boost Metabolism, *137*
Lemon Balm Blend to Banish Brain Fog, *138*
Lemon Peppermint Blend for Improved Digestion, *136*
Memory-Boosting Tea, *172–73*
Nettle Dandelion Blend for Liver Detox, *137*
tea ritual to promote happiness, *178–79*
Tea tree oil, magical and wellness properties, 34–35
Thyme, magical and wellness properties, 30–31
Tiger's eye, magical and wellness properties, 32–33
Tinctures, magical, 112–17. *See also* Herbal potions
Tools, 29–38. *See also* Candles; Crystals; Herbs
V
Valerian, magical and wellness properties, 30–31
Vetiver oil, magical and wellness properties, 34–35
W
Water, connecting with, *225–26*
Water element, connecting with, *92–93*
Water scrying, revealing unseen truths with, *187–88*
Weight, normalizing, 31
White, qualities associated with, 37
Wounds, healing, 31, 35, *122*
Y
Yarrow, magical and wellness properties, 30–31
Yellow, qualities associated with, 37
Ylang-ylang oil, magical and wellness properties, 34–35

About the Author

Krystle L. Jordan is a wellness writer who is certified in holistic nutrition and has been a practitioner of the craft for more than twenty years. An absolute lover of the earth and a part-time forest fairy, she focuses on living a sustainable, natural lifestyle and believes that everything carries its own energy and magic. Krystle has additional training in herbalism and body detoxification and is the creator of *The Wholesome Witch*. Find more of her work at TheWholesomeWitch.com.